THE MIRACLE IN ALOE VERA: THE FACTS ABOUT POLYMANNANS

Dr. Neecie Moore

CHARIS PUBLISHING CO.

A Charis Publishing Book

Published by Charis Publishing Co.
PO Box 740607
Dallas, Texas 75374

Cover by Mat Hames
Photography by Mickey Torres

Printed in the United States of America.

ISBN: 0-9647546-1-4

Dr. Neecie Moore
The Miracle in Aloe Vera
The Facts about Polymannans
Second Edition
$12.95 Softcover

In Loving Memory
of

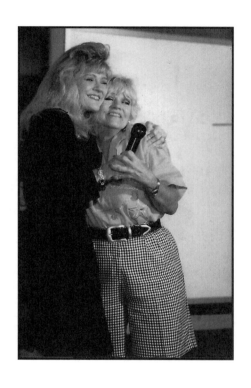

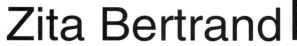

Zita Bertrand

DEDICATION

This book is dedicated to my mom and dad,
Red and Sissie Moore.

Heaven must have known that I would
need two very special parents,
and special people is what they are.

My dad delighted me with his
sense of humor and fun all my life.
We fished, fought with rolled up newspapers,
and made "horse faces" together for years.
He had a train put in a park in
Victoria, Texas, in his honor
and he also caught the
world's largest crab,
erected on Gaido's Restaurant
in Galveston, Texas.
(He also owns George Strait's
ocean front property in Arizona).

My mom is the most precious
of all God's angels.
Her prayers, her love, and her
devotion have kept me through all
my successes, and all my failures.
Her gentle words of encouragement
and her "Tender Touch"
have made me the most blessed
of little girls, teenagers, and
women.

I LOVE YOU BOTH!

ACKNOWLEDGEMENTS

I WOULD LIKE TO EXPRESS MY HEARTFELT THANKS TO ALL MY FRIENDS, FAMILY MEMBERS AND CLIENTS WHO ARE SO DEAR TO ME. AND ALSO TO:

KAY JACKSON, better known as K.K., who is the most precious friend, clinical assistant, and traveling partner anyone could ever have…I love you dearly;

DR. YOSAF HULGUS, who delights us by his very presence in our office;

KIMBERLY PARKER, who administrates the publishing company with such meticulous care, and is the greatest niece on earth… and to "Roger" for loving her and taking care of her;

DENNIS AND PATTY CROSS, for being such great partners and friends, and for housing me through transition times;

BRENT BOULDIN, my dear cousin, for all the faxes filled with news and encouragement; and all the help on my new endeavor;

PAT AND GLEN, CAROL AND ANDY, JANIS AND SKIP, "MOMSY," ASHLEY AND DICK, for being such a terrific family;

DR. REG MCDANIEL for helping me understand the mysteries of Aloe vera and for reviewing my manuscript;

GARY WATSON for countless hours of reviewing manuscripts, and holding on to those special keys, when a real Prince Charming wouldn't have even done it;

BILL & DONNA FIORETTI for making some impossible tasks possible for me – I could never thank you enough;

SAM & LINDA CASTER for being good friends and praying for me;

RAY ROBBINS, LARRY & JUDY, LOWELL & SHIRLEY, DOUG & ADRIEN, LUIS, CHIN LEE, BUTCH JOHNSON, TERRY, RON AND PAULETTE... and the countless others who have made being on the road so much fun;

MY "FRISTERS": ANITA, GINNY, MARY ELLEN, SHARI AND SUSAN for always being on my side and by my side;

JOEL JACKSON for delighting our office with his presence every day after school;

ALL MY NEIGHBORS: DONNA & BILL, DAVID & LESLIE, THE WILSONS, and all the folks in Branch, Texas, who so warmly welcomed me into their community;

THE PAP SQUAD, a cancer support group in Baton Rouge, LA, who bring hope and comfort to each other and their families (including mine);

JAMILLE AND TINA; CINDI, EDDIE, SHANE, AND SHANNA; AUNTIE HELEN AND SHARON K. for making the family reunion so much fun, and for being my family... I miss you all and love you so much; and to GEORGE AND DOROTHY MURRY for putting our reunion together;

MY SISTER, RUANA GRACE, for being my closest and dearest friend;

MY BUSHKA, REBEKAH GRACE, for bringing so much joy to my life;

MY NEPHEW, PAUL GRACE, who just can't beat me at "spit;" MY NEPHEW, JASON JONES, for taking such excellent care of our little home on the range, and just for being so wonderful;

DR. CHUCK "C.A." "TEX" KERIN for taking such great care of my animals and introducing me to two of the most delightful little girls I know: STEPHANIE AND KATHLEEN;

MY PRECIOUS GIRLS: TWYLA; JILL AND SARAH HOLT; and ANDREA, KELLI, AND COLLEEN HOLT, for all the fun, all the laughs, and all the love!

TABLE OF CONTENTS

SPECIAL NOTE

This book is for reference purposes and is not meant to be nor to replace medical advice. The information and material presented is strictly intended for educational purposes. Neither the publishers nor the author are intending to make recommendations about your health care. The purpose of this book is not for self-diagnosis nor self-treatment of any illness or disease. Before making changes in your diet, your medication or your exercise program, consult with your physician.

1

THE HISTORY OF ALOE VERA

In 1935, a Maryland physician, Dr. C.E. Collins, had a 31-year-old female with severe skin damage from radiation treatments. A skin graft to treat the burned areas of her skin had been recommended. Instead, having heard of successful treatment of skin damage with Aloe vera, Dr. Collins tried fresh Aloe. The affected area was healed in 36 days.

A radically new medical phenomenon? One that has since transformed treatment of burns and other skin disorders? Comically...tragically...the answer is definitely "no" to both questions. Aloe was neither new then, nor has it been universally accepted as a skin treatment.

The story of Aloe vera is both ancient and new, both science and fraud, both tremendous success and dismal failure. But as you will see, enlightenment is rapidly coming to the mystery of this ancient medicinal plant.

EARLIEST RECORDED USES OF ALOE VERA

The saying "older than Methuselah" is certainly a phrase that applies to the uses of Aloe vera. Since the earliest recorded medical history, Aloe vera has been used in the healing process. The Hindus believe that the plant was brought to us from the Garden of Eden at the beginning of time (Coats, 1984). The first known recorded medical uses of Aloe vera were inscribed on clay tablets in 2100 B.C. by a Sumerian physician in an early Mesopotamian civilization, although the tablets were not excavated until 4,000 years later and were not translated until 1953 (Danhof, 1987).

Around 1550 B.C., the Egyptians listed herbal plants for medicinal purposes in their famous Ebers Papyrus, and Aloe was one of the cathartics listed. The papers listed 12 formulas for the medicinal uses of Aloe (Hennessee, 1989). By 600 B.C., the Arabs were experts at using Aloe, using it mostly for its laxative effect. In 25 B.C., Celcus also mentions Aloe and its use as a laxative in his *De Medicina*.

THE USES FOR ALOE VERA EXPAND

Not until 35 A.D. was there recorded medical history that indicated more extensive uses for Aloe. Pliny the Elder included various remedies using Aloe, such as prevention of hair loss, relief from headaches, healing diseases of the eye, healing bruises and other marks on the skin, healing tonsil and gum problems, stopping hemorrhaging, curing wounds, treating hemorrhoidal conditions, alleviating indigestion, and, of course, for laxative uses (Kent, 1979).

In 74 A.D., Dioscordes, a Roman pharmacist, in his *De Materia Medica* listed many medical uses for Aloe. Included in his list were medicinal properties such as healing wounds, repressing boils, healing bruises, eliminating skin abrasions, stopping hair loss, soothing eye sores, healing genital ulcers, ameliorating tonsilitis, healing hemorrhoids, and, of course, relieving constipation or bowel problems by acting as a laxative (Coats, 1984).

In 625 A.D. and halfway around the world, the Chinese began recording their uses of Aloe vera. Li Sun mentions using it to treat sinuosities and to reduce fever in children (Danhof, 1987). In 685 A.D., Paul of Aegina, a Greek surgeon, described using Aloe as an anti-inflammatory agent, as well as a healing agent for ulcers (Kent, C.M.1979). In 980 A.D., Avicenna began understanding that the Socotrine Aloes were superior to the Arabian Aloes, and recorded the many uses of Aloe in his *Cannon of Medicine.*

CONTROVERSY ABOUT ALOE VERA

During this same time period, controversy first

appeared about the use of Aloe. Mesue of Damascus noted that the use of Aloe as a purgative could result in abdominal cramping and nausea, and recommended the use of milder substances (Kent, C.M. 1979). This was the beginning of the controversy that has followed Aloe from Mesue's time until today.

In 1492, during his famous voyage, Columbus, wrote about what he saw in the New World in his journal, "...I arrived here at the Cape of the Islet and anchored... Here I came upon Aloes and tomorrow I have decided to take 10 quintals of it, for they tell me it is worth much." (Morison, 1963, 77).

In 1563, a Portuguese physician wrote about his findings of botanicals that he gathered while traveling extensively in India. He wrote about Aloe's effectiveness in treating bladder and kidney disease, pain, and in relieving inflammation (Danhof, 1987).

By the early 1700s, Aloe was in vogue. It became fashionable to grow Aloe plants in decorative pots on terraces and balconies, (Kent, 1979). By the mid 1700s, medicines concocted using Aloe were quite numerous. In the *Pharmacopeia* of the Royal College of Medicine of London, at least nine of the major medicinal mixtures contained Aloe (Danhof, 1987).

In the early 1800s, Dr. Quallame Olivier, of India, reportedly began to use Aloe to induce pregnancy in infertile women and to use it to regulate menstrual cycles. At the same time, northern Europeans were making a tonic of Aloe to treat consumption, a fatally chronic disease (Coats, 1984). In 1851, the first chemical compound extracted from the Aloe plant was identified as aloin. Aloin is the black and brown substance with the bitter taste in Aloe (Coats, 1984).

ALOE VERA AS STUDIED BY THE MILITARY

Early in the 1900s, Sir George Watt used Aloe extensively to treat the various needs of the British troops stationed in India. Among the conditions he listed in his *Dictionary of the Economic Products of India (1908)* that Aloe could treat were irregular menstruation, headaches, hysteria, constipation, bronchial conditions, sprains and contusions, diseases of the spleen, hair dye, stimulation of hair growth, brain diseases, hemorrhoids, eye conditions, colic, pneumonia, gonorrhea, and rheumatism (Danhof, 1987).

At the same time Dr. Collins successfully treated the radiation burn case described earlier, Dr. Crewe (1937) published an article listing the various external uses of Aloe. He included the treatment of chronic ulcers, thermal burns, eczema, scalds, sunburns, minor injuries, poison ivy, and itching around the female genital areas.

THE SEARCH FOR THE ACTIVE INGREDIENT

In the late 1930s, the first serious, scientific attempt to identify the active ingredient in Aloe vera was published (Rowe & Parks, 1939). This study, and many that followed, failed to isolate the specific active ingredient(s) responsible for the plant's medicinal benefits. This failure followed the Aloe plant for another 50 years.

However, like many mysteries of life and medicine, clues as to the location of the right path began to surface. At the end of the path was the identification of the active ingredient in Aloe, and most important, why the application of Aloe seemed to be so erratic in its effect.

Research conducted in the 1950s set the stage. Ikawa and Niemann (1951) began isolating compounds in Aloe. They determined that the Aloe gel consisted of muco-polysaccharides (glucose, mannose, uronic acid, and rhamnose). The Niemann work was basic research, intended to simply discover what was present. Although analytical chemistry is not of particular interest to a layman, the major contribution of this work was that there active ingredients in Aloe, and that further study was definitely needed.

The first sign, "This Is the Way!" had been tacked to a tree on the right path.

2

THE MIRACLE IN ALOE UNFOLDS: AN ACTIVE INGREDIENT

For centuries, people of various cultures, countries, and backgrounds have turned to plants for their healing properties, seeking remedies for ailments of all kinds. However, modern medicine, as practiced in the United States and most of western civilization, takes a disdainful and arrogant attitude toward the healing compounds found naturally existing in plants, compounds that are not "synthesized by man." This attitude is pervasive in the halls of medicine, of the pharmaceutical companies, and of the FDA. An article in the *Houston Chronicle* in 1992 exposed this attitude by stating: "…in the United States, pharmaceutical researchers have shown only an on-again, off-again interest in investigating plants' curative properties" (Beachy, 1992). Only recently has "modern" medicine been dragged, kicking and screaming, to the cutting edge of pharmacology: plants.

CONTROVERSY OVER ALOE'S EFFECTIVENESS

Of all the plant-medicine storehouses, Aloe has been

one of the most controversial. The reason for this controversy was the maddening inconsistency of results. One clinician would report great results, another would get nothing. The fact that traditional medicine would be cautious about Aloe is understandable, given the attitude about "natural" or "plant" medicines in the modern era.

Through a long series of events, however, the mystery of widely varying results from Aloe treatments has largely been solved. One of the early steps came as a result of the military's need to combat radiation burns in the 1950s. Federal research dollars supported a project at the Radiation Burn Center of Los Alamos, sponsored by the U.S. Atomic Energy Commission. Dr. Lushbaugh and Dr. Hale (1953) were in charge of this project to study the healing of Beta radiation burn wounds. Rabbits were exposed to Beta radiation, causing burn wounds. Researchers then treated two of the wounds on the belly of each rabbit with freshly harvested Aloe vera. They treated two other wounds on the rabbit's belly with a commercially prepared Aloe vera product. The remaining two wounds on each rabbit's belly remained untreated. The wounds treated with freshly harvested Aloe vera were healed within two months, much quicker than the commercially prepared Aloe vera. The findings were quite significant, indicating there was an active ingredient in the freshly harvested Aloe vera which was lost during processing, or with time, when stored.

Several years later (1957) under the auspices of the U.S. Army, six patients who had second and third degree burns on their legs were studied. No differences were found between those treated with Aloe vera ointment and those treated with other medication. Nine patients with skin cancer who had received radiation burns from their treatments were studied. No difference in healing time were noticed between those treated with Aloe vera ointment and those treated with other ointments. The conclusions: "There would seem to be no indication to use Aloe vera in presently available forms for mass treatment of thermal or radiation burns." (Ashley et al., 1957).

RESEARCH PRODUCES PUZZLING, MIXED RESULTS

Although the results were mixed (over such a widely divergent range of maladies, how could it have been otherwise), the results for burn wound healing were sufficiently positive for the FDA to issue the following response that, "the ointment does actually regenerate skin tissue" (Flagg, 1959, 27). This was a major breakthrough in the Aloe industry.

Both sides of the research controversy were being conducted and reported by reputable sources (McDaniel, 1994). The mixed reports were confusing to the medical and lay communities alike. Clearly, there were benefits from Aloe; however, "whatever medicinal properties rested in the plant could neither be deciphered nor borne out in the labs" (Coats, 1984, 23).

Critics of Aloe capitalized on the anecdotal claims and exaggerations being made by promoters of totally fraudulent products. Unfounded claims in promotional literature have not been helpful to those attempting to substantiate the medicinal value of Aloe. One critic stated that Aloe was "almost as effective as baptismal water, but infinitely more expensive" (Gjerstad, 1969). The promoters, seizing on the mystery of Aloe, sold all manner of products. Products were sold that "contain 100% Aloe vera," "is made with 100% Aloe vera," "is derived from 100% Aloe vera," and on and on. Most of these products labeled "Aloe" were quite useless, and analysis disclosed no plant-source molecules. At the same time, honest and dedicated people were growing the plant and continuing to make great progress due to their experience of success.

As the number of worthless products increased, the FDA became increasingly active in its enforcement actions against these products. In 1981, the Aloe industry was almost shut down because the FDA stated that 90 percent of the Aloe sold in the United States was fraudulent (McDaniel, 1994).

WHY SOME ALOE HAS NO MEDICINAL VALUE

There are many reasons why much of the Aloe being sold has no medicinal value. For example, to eliminate the bitter taste of Aloe, some companies filter the plant through charcoal. Although this process eliminates the bitter taste, it also removes the active ingredients (McDaniel, 1994). Coats (1984) lists additional reasons why the Aloe isn't always effective, including use of the wrong species of the plant, use of immature plants, use of leaves from dehydrated plants, and erratic or improper use of the plant.

From within the Aloe industry, a new organization was formed in an attempt to save the industry: the International Aloe Science Council. The Council began a major crusade to maintain integrity and eliminate fraudulent products from the market. The Council adopted a certification program for Aloe products, and for Aloe-containing products (Pelley, 1992).

After years of effort, some progress has been observed. Dr. Pelley of the University of Texas Medical Branch in Galveston, Texas, presented the results of his analytical survey of Aloe products at a 1994 conference in Dallas. He stated that the fraudulent Aloe product rate had been reduced to 70 percent (McDaniel, 1994). Although the Council has had some success, it has had its own internal battles, and there have been, and continue to be, sharp differences about various Aloe products and claims. The Council has been effective in helping to eliminate some of the more egregious marketing frauds, and urges its members to conform to FDA regulations relating to making medical claims for this natural, non-drug plant gel.

THE IMPORTANCE OF THE PROCESSING OF ALOE

A 1981 study by W.D. Winters and others at the University of Texas at San Antonio Department of Microbiology, found that the biogenic stimulation ability of Aloe vera can be reduced or even reversed by improper processing. As Winters points out in his report, in vitro studies (outside the body) can eliminate some of the countless variables present during in vivo (in the body) studies. The detailed analysis of cell cultures studied by Winters and his associates showed properly prepared Aloe was effective in promoting healing at the cell level.

However, critics continued to ridicule Aloe, scoffing at the notion that proper handling of the plant made for effective healing compounds, insisting there was no medicinal value in the Aloe plant. Two critics remarked: "The question logically arises why some larger research or pharmaceutical company has not followed up on this apparently valuable medical agent" (Gjerstad and Riner, 1968).

For whatever reasons, products containing Aloe vera were sometimes effective, sometimes ineffective. The state of the Aloe industry was summarized well by two authors: "The 'scientific' evidence for its rejection is almost countered by the 'scientific' evidence for its beneficial properties" (Grindlay and Reynolds, 1986). Many in the scientific community were interested in the exact nature of the difference in those products that were effective and those that were ineffective.

THE SEARCH FOR AN ACTIVE INGREDIENT
CONTINUES

One of those interested in Aloe research was Bill McAnalley, Ph.D., who in 1979 was working on his doctoral degree in pharmacology at the University of Texas Health

Science Center in Dallas, Texas. With some funding from an entrepreneur who owned a cosmetic and natural foods business, McAnalley began studies to determine the medicinal benefits (or lack of benefits) of Aloe vera.

Very quickly, research indicated that the gel of the Aloe plant, when applied soon after cutting the plant, facilitated the healing of wounds. It was apparent that there was indeed medicinal value, but that the value was dependent on the time since the harvesting of the Aloe vera leaf.

McAnalley's research indicated that when the Aloe plant is cut or compressed, an enzyme is released. When this enzyme is released, it begins to destroy those active ingredient(s) which are of therapeutic value. This "determined the basis for disagreements over the presence of a medically beneficial principal in the gel of the Aloe vera plant. Investigators with conflicting results could both be correct even though one reported no benefit and another reported a medical benefit attributed to the use of Aloe vera "gel" (McDaniel et al., 1994).

McAnalley (1988), as director of research for Carrington Laboratories, Inc. in Irving, Texas, developed and patented a process for deactivating the destructive enzymes. Once the enzymes were deactivated, processed Aloe vera had a shelf-life. The freeze-dried dehydration process produces a purified powdered extract from the clear gel center of the Aloe leaf that contains the medicinally active ingredients of fresh Aloe.

At the same time, McAnalley also successfully identified and extracted the active chemical substance, and found a means to stabilize the active ingredient. He found the active ingredient to be a polysaccharide. More specifically, a mucilaginous polysaccharide.

A MUCILAGINOUS POLYSACCHARIDE EXPLAINED

To those outside the biochemical scientific field, mucilaginous polysaccharide are just two words that are difficult to pronounce and have no meaning. To simplify, they indicate a chemical structure consisting of a long chain of sugars linked together to form a starch. The functional component of Aloe is a complex starch and is also referred to as a B-(1,4)-linked mannan. Such biological molecules are classified as carbohydrates. The Aloe mannans were given the trade name of *acemannan* by the United States Adopted Names Council of the American Medical Association. Acemannan has come to be used as the designation for an unapproved drug by the FDA regulatory process. Manapol™ is defined as a nutritional supplement. Those B-(1,4) mannan chains unique to the Aloe plant can be collectively termed "polymannans."

The importance of polymannans to the human body is phenomenal. In a benchmark paper, Tizard and a group of researchers noted that not only were these polymannans active, but they were also nontoxic (Tizard et al.,1989). These means that not only are there tremendous benefits from the use of Aloe vera, but regardless of the dosage, there are no harmful side effects which are found in most prescribed medicines.

To simplify how polymannans act in our body's biochemistry is a difficult task. A biochemist might find this explanation an oversimplification, but perhaps it will aid in understanding the capabilities of the active ingredient, the polymannans, of Aloe vera once it enters the human body.

When polymannans enter the body, they are bound to a receptor site. These receptor sites are on the cell membrane structure of our cells. Once bound to a receptor site, they activate macrophages and other cells of the immune system (Hasenclever and Mitchell, 1964). Macrophages are among the cells that control our immune system. They wander throughout the body to monitor tissue for damage, dysfunction, infection, malignant change, and other defective conditions. When the macrophages find something abnormal, they call for a cellular defense team by activating messenger molecules. These messengers are called cytokines. The cytokines then initiate and induce an immune response to counteract whatever specific disease condition is affecting the body.

Interestingly, these cytokines are released in the exact precise amount needed to combat whatever disease is present. When these cytokines are given synthetically, the dosage is uncertain, and overdose with serious side effects can occur. However, when natural B-(1,4)-linked mannans, as occurring naturally in Aloe vera, are ingested, some mechanism in our body determines the necessary level of macrophages, and deactivates the synthesis and secretion once the necessary amount to combat the disease is achieved. It "enhances, rather than overrides this [immune] system." (Carrington Labs,

1993). This creates a situation where even high doses of polymannans have been repeatedly shown to be nontoxic (Ray Dirks Research, 1992).

One of the unique properties of a polymannan is that it is not broken down in the digestive system. Other polysaccharides of different sugars and different linkages, such as starch from corn, are used as an energy source or fuel. Therefore, these polymannans (from the aloe) are preserved until they are absorbed from the digestive tract and are delivered to the cell. In summation, these polymannans activate the normal mechanisms of healing when it is needed, where it is needed, and in the correct amount that it is needed in response to any abnormal cells or damaged tissue in the body. This is why the polymannans show promise in addressing a wide range of diseases and conditions, including canker sores, hay fever, wound care, cancer, AIDS, and ulcerative colitis (Carrington Laboratories, Inc., 1993).

B-(1,4)-LINKED MANNANS, MANAPOL, AND ACEMANNAN

Carrington Laboratories now holds 56 patents regarding these polymannans. The patents include composition of matter, processing, and use patents, covering 21 different countries. While the United States Adopted Names Council of the American Medical Association has issued the name acemannan to the B-(1,4)-linked mannans, Carrington obtained the trademark name "Manapol" for its specific B-

(1,4)-linked mannan.

There is a difference between acemannan and Manapol. Manapol is the first pass, freeze-dried extract of fresh Aloe, the raw material from which acemannan can be produced. Manapol contains at least 56 percent polymannans, while acemannan contains at least 86 to 93 percent. Manapol is actually a nutritional supplement conforming to FDA regulations for food processing that contains the polymannans that stimulate the immune system.

These polymannans have powerful implications for the health of our nation. "From 1985 to 1993, Dr. McAnalley and Dr. McDaniel, together with other scientists, conducted a series of studies demonstrating the benefits of acemannan on over 100 different disease conditions" (Pullin, 1994). Further research may bring other chemicals from Aloe to the forefront of plant medicines. As pointed out by Davis et. al. (1991, 475), "In fact, one tablespoon of Aloe vera contains over 75 different chemicals that have biological activity."

STANDARDIZED TESTING FOR PRODUCTS CONTAINING ALOE

One of the most important aspects of progressive Aloe research is the development of a standardized test. As pointed out by Hennessee and Cook, "As long as promoters continue to sell colorless, tasteless, odorless, and therefore medically useless products, the need for standardized testing is imperative" (1989, 52). Researchers at Texas A&M used high pressure liquid chromatography (HPLC) to determine a chromatographic "profile"— a distinctive, reproducible, graphic pattern, more distinctive than a human fingerprint, that can prove the presence of Aloe. The analysis is centered on the presence of soluble solids. The researchers found the profile presented a high peak at the front of the profile, followed by several lower peaks. To a layman, the high peak seems more impressive, but the researchers pointed out that it is the distinctive pattern that includes the presence of smaller peaks that is actually of significance. The high peak is present in several other plants, including some Easter lilies and ferns. The researchers stated that the presence of a unique family of peaks, each signifying the presence of unique phytochemicals, was necessary to confirm the presence of Aloe. The use of HPLC and its results has spawned some controversy in the Aloe industry because analysis of some commercially successful products made by dedicated, honest Aloe products manufacturers have shown them to contain little or no active polymannans from Aloe. Naturally the makers of these products wish to discredit the method of analysis. However, it is clear that HPLC is currently the best method for determining the presence of polymannans and to prove that gel from the Aloe plant is actually in the product.

From years of folklore to current medical research, Aloe vera has been shown to be a powerful remedy and a powerful preventative. Finally, we can know that content standardization and procedures are being developed to insure that products on the market will produce the health and healing benefits that have sustained folk use of Aloe for over 5,000 years.

3

WOUND CARE AND HEALING: THE IMPACT OF ALOE VERA

All of us from time to time experience wounding in one form or another. In the United States, physicians in emergency rooms around the country treat over 10 million traumatic wounds annually. Wounds have been treated with a variety of methods and remedies through the years, with such things as mud packs, honey poultices, fire, dry dressings, and moist dressings (McAnalley et al., 1994).

The word "wound" has many implications and encompasses a wide variety of conditions. Mosby's Medical Dictionary (1990) defines a wound as "any physical injury involving a break in the skin, usually caused by an act or accident rather than by a disease." In a patent for a wound cleanser, McAnalley et al., (1994) defined a wound as a physical or chemical trauma to the body or a traumatic insult to the integrity of tissue. Danhof (1987) included these conditions in a list of wounds: insect bites, burns, scalds, chronic ulcers, abrasions, bruises, contusions, cuts, lacerations, and blisters.

ALOE AS AGE OLD WOUND HEALER

With the many conditions to which we apply the word "wound," one thing is constant. Through the ages, people of all cultures have used Aloe vera to promote healing of their wounds (Coats, 1984). One writer stated that the "beneficial effects attributed to Aloe in the process of wound care are so miraculous as to seem more like myth than fact" (Heggers, 1991). However, there is, in recent times, more scientific data from which to judge the benefits of Aloe in wound care. The results of this scientific data and of scientific studies indicate that "Aloe is, as recorded in ancient manuscripts, a drug of enormous therapeutic potential" (Heggers, 1991).

Historically, there have been numerous claims about the benefits of Aloe used to treat wounds. Pliny used Aloe to treat the wounds associated with leprosy (Hennessee and Cook, 1989). In his First Century text, *De Materia Medica,* Dioscordes claimed that Aloe healed wounds by conglutination [congealing]. Aloe was used extensively in South Africa to heal wounds resulting from battle or from hunting (Coats, 1984). Veterinarians have used Aloe to treat animal wounds for many years, and have written extensively about those results ("The Local Action of Aloes on Regeneration," 1941).

The scientific data regarding wound healing is difficult to address for many reasons. One reason is the vast difference of definitions of the word "healing." Another is the need in a scientific study for two similar wounds in the same subject so that one can be treated and the other used as a control.

However, when more than one subject is used, it is difficult to account for the differences in healing abilities of the individuals. Also, as already stated in an earlier chapter, the results vary depending on the time between the harvest of the Aloe vera plant and the time it is used in the study, once again emphasizing the importance of using Aloe vera that has been processed appropriately (Fulton, 1990).

It should be noted that the value of Aloe became controversial only in the modern era, when urbanization took people away from fresh plants. Aloe applied immediately has the best chance of being effective. Aloe harvested and stored, if not done properly, is useless.

WOUND HEALING

Wound healing is a "complex cascade of biochemical and cellular events designed to achieve restoration of tissue integrity following injury" (Barbul, 1990, 433). For wounds to heal with maximum efficiency, it is imperative that proper cleansing is done to prevent the development of infection and to promote healing of the tissue injured in the wounding process. This requires the removal of all contaminating bacteria and other foreign material from the wound. One of the problems with this important step has been the kinds of cleansers commercially available. Many of these agents cause further damage to the tissue, resulting in further wounding (Johnson et al., 1989).

IF IT'S SAFE FOR YOUR EYES, IT'S SAFE FOR YOUR WOUNDS

In the process of inventing an Aloe vera product suitable for wound cleansing, McAnalley (1994) used the eye test as a standard: "Don't put in a wound what you wouldn't put in an eye." To conduct this test for suitability, he put his Aloe wound cleansing formula into one of each of the eyes of six rabbits. Although three of the rabbits had a slight discharge from the treated eye within one hour of the application, all rabbits had clear eyes at 24-, 48-, and 72-hour readings. Additional studies indicate that the commercial Aloe vera wound dressing developed by Drs. McAnnalley and McDaniel (Carrington Dermal Wound Gel) did no further damage to the injured tissue when used as a cleanser, and actually stimulated the cell replication necessary for wound repair (Johnson et al., 1989), Therefore, Aloe vera products were demonstrated to be suited not only for the healing of wounds, but also for the cleansing of wounds. Attesting to the effectiveness of this philosophy, Carrington's wound care division grew to $25 million in annual sales in 10 years with virtually no advertising, few published papers, and a tiny sales force. Word-of-mouth in the medical community did the selling.

THE JOB OF MACROPHAGES IN WOUND HEALING

When a wound occurs, additional macrophages

migrate into the site of the wound within 48 to 96 hours. These macrophages participate in the inflammatory and debridement (self-cleansing) stages, and continue their work in the fibroblastic phase (where the tissue begins to bind together and heal). The macrophages then send messages that continue the fibroblastic replication, which then leads to remodeling and improvement in the wounded area (Barbul, 1990). "Cells in a wound communicate with each other through substances known as growth factors. Growth factors are polypeptide hormones that are stored by most cells and are secreted into local tissues. Once the growth factor has been attracted to the wound area, it binds to a cell surface receptor, usually a fibroblast. This sequence initiates the biological response, wound healing" (Davis, 1994). Earlier discussions of how the polymannans activate and work effectively with the macrophage system substantiate the importance of Aloe in wound healing. Dr. Davis, a researcher at the Pennsylvania College of Podiatric Medicine, supported this theory by stating that "The 'Aloe Vera molecule' can stimulate the fibroblast to increase collagen and proteoglycans" (Davis, 1993, 8), both of which are essential to wound healing. It has also been stated that the "macrophage system orchestrates all phases of wound healing" (McAnalley et al., 1994).

STUDIES ABOUT ALOE AND WOUND HEALING

As early as 1967, studies were being conducted to determine the effectiveness of Aloe in the treatment of wounds. One study noted that abrasion wounds healed at least one-third faster when treated with Aloe vera (Barnes, 1967). In 1973, a study was conducted using Aloe vera gel to treat leg ulcers. This study was particularly interesting because leg ulcers are prone to resist treatment due to poor blood circulation, resulting in a challenge to physicians treating them. In this study, the leg ulcers treated with the Aloe gel indicated that it had a stimulating effect on healing the ulcers. The same study also found that Aloe vera was beneficial in the treatment of acne (Zawahry et al., 1973, 72). As a result of this study, the researchers stated: "We believe that the active principal for promoting healing is mucopolysaccharides which are present in high concentration in Aloe gel."

A 1987 (Davis, 67) study of wounded mice and rats found Aloe to be effective in wound treatment. The researchers found that RNA and vitamin C did not add to the effectiveness of Aloe. "Within the Aloe vera treated mice and rat groups, an increase in skin [blood] circulation was observed with redness in the wounded area. Aloe also seems to continue its effectiveness even after wound closure by avoiding contracture and hypertropic scarring."

In 1989, a study was conducted using mice as subjects. Mice with wounds were divided into groups. Each mouse received a wound on its back. One group received Aloe vera orally, another group received Aloe vera in a cream form. The final group received no treatment. It was noted that wounds treated orally and topically with Aloe vera were reduced significantly, indicating that both means of administration are effective (Davis et al., 1989).

ALOE AS A TREATMENT FOR ACNE

In 1990, a study was performed on the effectiveness of Aloe vera on acne lesions. Eighteen patients were used for the study, each receiving Aloe vera treatment to one side of their face, and a standard wound dressing on the other. Within 24 to 48 hours, swelling was reduced where Aloe had been applied. Within three to four days there was less pussiness and crusting on the side receiving Aloe treatment. In five to six days, healing of the wound was complete. The healing occurred at least 72 hours quicker on the side of the face to which the Aloe vera was applied (Fulton, 1990).

POLYMANNANS AS WOUND HEALERS

Studies have been conducted to specifically assess the benefits of the polymannans to wound healing. One such study employed fifteen dogs with paw injuries. Twelve of the dogs received the treatment of a triple antibiotic cream to one paw, and the treatment of a polymannan wound gel to the other. Three of the dogs received no treatment to either paw. The dogs were observed at intervals of 7, 14, and 21 days. Although the end results of healing were the same, the paws treated with the polymannan gel demonstrated more healing within seven days. This opened new doors, suggesting that perhaps the polymannans might be effective in treatment of wounds that were slow to heal or treatment resistant due to innate physical abuse, i.e., pads of an animal's paw. (Swaim et al., 1992). In additional studies using mice and guinea pigs for subjects, it was noted that the polymannans also promoted faster reconnection of tissue when compared to control wounds (Tizard, 1992). Further studies indicated that when guinea pigs were given four different kinds of wounds, the polymannans accelerated healing in three of the four different types of wounds (Parnell & Tizard, 1992).

Carrington Laboratories has developed several products for wound care. Their wound gel "is approved for use is all stage of decubitus ulcers, stasis ulcers, first and second degree burns, cuts, abrasions, skin irritations and peristomal care" (Carrington Laboratories, March 1993).

Indeed the effectiveness of Aloe vera, specifically the polymannans, is well researched and documented. As the search continues for more sophisticated pharmaceuticals to treat wounds, ancient Aloe remains an available, natural, sure adjuvant to wound healing.

4

ANTI-INFLAMMATORY DISEASE AND ALOE AS AN ANTI-INFLAMMATORY

Inflammation is closely related to wound healing, because inflammation is a part of the wounding process and the healing of the wound. *Mosby's Medical Dictionary (1990)* defines inflammation as "the protective response of the tissues of the body to irritation to injury. Its cardinal signs are redness, heat, swelling, and pain, accompanied by loss of function." The term inflammation can encompass everything from uncomplicated postoperative swelling to crippling rheumatoid arthritis (Davis et al., 1989). Inflammation disorders include many maladies of a variety of causes such as Graves' disease, lupus, connective tissue disease, polymyositis, dermatomyositis, and scleroderma, just to name a few.

Inflammation is not solely the result of direct physical wounding. Annually, we are exposed to 60,000 chemical pollutants and 200 radioactive toxins which can cause severe inflammation, infections, and internal or external pain (Schechter, 1994). Toxins, improper diet, some medication, excessive exposure to the sun, and leakage of implanted silicone breast enlargements are among other causes of inflammatory disorders. Inflammation is actually a defensive response in reaction to any injury arising from trauma to our tissue or cells (Sener & Bingol, 1988). Although inflammation is vital to the healing process, if it is uncontrolled or if it persists, it can lead to serious conditions (Davis et al., 1991).

Inflammation occurs in tissue that has been traumatized due to the release of chemical mediators which aggravate the inflammatory process (Davis et al., 1991). Two of the chemical mediators produced in a wounded area are bradykinin and histamine. Bradykinin is one of the most potent pain-producing agents (Obata, 1991). Degrading the bradykinin not only relieves pain, but also relieves inflammation. Aloe vera is effective as an anti-inflammatory because of its ability to block these chemical mediators, ameliorating the symptoms (Obata, 1991; Davis et al., 1991; Fujita et al., 1976). Exactly how and why this chemical reaction occurs in the presence of Aloe vera has been the topic of many studies. One belief is that the amino acid components in Aloe vera, phenylalanine and tryptophan, which are known to have anti-inflammatory activity, are the reason for the anti-inflammatory effects in Aloe vera (Davis et al., 1991).

ALOE'S ANTI-INFLAMMATORY PROPERTIES

Aloe vera not only has anti-inflammatory properties, but when administered over a progressive time interval, there is a proportionate increase in anti-inflammatory activity (Davis et al., 1989). In recent studies (Davis et al., 1994), mannose-6-phosphate was isolated from the polysaccharide chain in Aloe vera. When treating ear inflammation of mice, it was found that the mannose-6-phosphate reduced inflammation and promoted healing.

In another research project, mice and rats were used to determine the effectiveness of Aloe vera, and of Aloe vera combined with hydrocortisone to treat inflammation. When Aloe vera was used adjuvantly with hydrocortisone, ear swelling in adult female mice demonstrated a 97 percent reduction. When the Aloe and hydrocortisone mixture was administered to adult male rats with paw wounds, there was an 88.1 percent reduction in the swelling. The results indicated Aloe complemented the steroid while reducing its normal toxic effects (Davis et al., 1991).

THE SIGNIFICANCE OF A NEW ANTI-INFLAMMATORY AGENT

This finding was of great significance because of the need for "an effective, specific, and relatively nontoxic anti-inflammatory compound... for patients with inflammation disorders" (Davis et al., 1989). Previously, there have been two groups of drugs used as anti-inflammatories. One was the nonsteroidal aspirin-like compounds. However, these compounds provide only symptomatic relief and do not halt the progression of injury to the tissue. In addition, these compounds have been known to cause gastric disorders and ulceration of the intestinal tract with prolonged use. In large doses, aspirin has caused death. The second group was the anti-inflammatory corticosteroids. These steroids have toxic effects inducing diabetes, osteoporosis, cataracts, psychosis, and serious infections, which eliminates the ability to prolong the administration of them as an anti-inflammatory (Sener & Bingol, 1988).

ALOE AND ARTHRITIS

One of the most devastating forms of inflammation is arthritis. Millions of Americans have some form of this debilitating disease. Aloe has been shown to be effective in reducing the pain and swelling from arthritis. In a 1981 study, Hanley et al., induced arthritis in rats, then treated different groups of rats with either ascorbic acid, thymus extract, Aloe extract or DNA. "On day seven, with DNA, Aloe, and ascorbic acid, an early trend was noted toward inhibition of edema [swelling] in the non-injected paw. Only Aloe showed edema inhibition in the injected paw. However, by day 14, Aloe produced a pronounced inhibition in both paws. On day 21, Aloe produced the most radical edema reduction in both paws. Only Aloe showed a continued trend in edema reduction in both paws. Inhibition was 72 and 48 percent within the noninjected and injected paws, respectively."

LUPUS AND ALOE

Rita Thompson tells her courageous story about her battle with such drugs and a connective tissue disease, lupus, in her book: *Lupus, Aloe Vera, and Me* (1989). Rita tells her story of being misdiagnosed as having rheumatoid arthritis initially, then being rediagnosed when rashes appeared on her legs. They first appeared for a week or more, then disappeared, only to reappear more severely. As the outbreaks became worse, she was hospitalized numerous times. At one point, the outbreaks were so painful that she wore no clothes, but a plastic wrap that was lubricated with special ointments.

When Rita had lost all her hair, and even all her fingernails, one doctor proposed a last ditch effort—heavy doses of steroid drugs. In search of a humane treatment for her lupus, Rita discovered Aloe vera juice. Within a month, her symptoms of two and a half years diminished and her skin began clearing (Coats, 1984). Certainly for Rita Thompson, the results of using Aloe vera as an anti-inflammatory were miraculous.

On interviewing Dr. McDaniel while serving as a scientific consultant for Carrington Labs and Emprise International (now called Mannatech Incorporated), he stated that elimination of the discomforts and disabilities of lupus has been the most consistent improvement reported anecdotally . This includes reversal of progressive renal failure and improvements in patients with the "Lupus-like Syndrome" of silicon breast implants. "I am amazed at the healing capacity of the human body if we provide nutritionally (that is we provide the complex starch from the Aloe plant and Dioscorea from the yam) what the innate biochemistry needs to work with, available through our diet," he stated.

5

THE USE OF ALOE VERA IN THE TREATMENT OF BURNS

Burns are a major source of trauma and a source that expands as we are exposed more and more to burning agents in our everyday life. Compared to our forefathers whose lives were based in agriculture, we have an enormous number of possible burn sources: household chemicals, electrical wiring and appliances, and countless encounters with heat and with hot liquids. Our sophisticated industrial and manufacturing techniques expose us to thousands of burning agents.

ANCIENT USES OF ALOE IN BURN HEALING

Anecdotal evidence of Aloe's power to heal burns comes to us from as far back as Pliny the Elder in 35 A.D. (Kent, 1979). In the centuries since, the Earth's peoples, from the Chinese to the Egyptians to the Indians of Central America, have used fresh Aloe leaves to help heal burns.

The care and treatment of burns is intensely studied because the healing process has been found to be very complicated. Much trial and error has occurred over the years, and today the healing pathway is still not well known. As with many medical treatments, researchers observe a mode of treatment that works, then try to determine why it works.

So it has been with Aloe and burn healing. Scientists could not help but pay attention to the mountain of folklore about Aloe's healing power, including its effect on burns. Through the study of the mechanics and biochemistry of wound healing, along with the study of the chemical composition of Aloe, researchers have tried to match the healing pathway with the compounds known to exist in Aloe. In this manner, scientists have attempted to explain why (and most importantly, under what conditions) Aloe works.

HOW ALOE WORKS IN THE HEALING OF BURNS

One observation that several investigators (Kivett, 1989) have made is the high concentration in burn blisters of a biochemical substance called "thromboxane." Thromboxane is known as a potent vasoconstrictor (constricts vessels in the body), whereas its counterpart prostacycline has the opposite effect on vasculature. Therefore, these two substances balance each other to produce a balance in skin tissue (Heggers, 1985). Through a series of experiments, researchers determined that if they could inhibit the formation of thromboxane at the burn site, the usual continuation of injury to the site that normally occurs is reversed. The studies indicated that dermal microcirculation, the blood circulation in microscopic capillaries in the skin, was preserved if thromboxane formation could be reduced at the burn site (Heggers, 1985). In preventing thromboxane response, blood cells are prevented from sticking to vessel walls, and vessels dilate, allowing improved blood circulation.

Aloe inhibits the production of the enzyme that is needed to produce thromboxane (Heggers, 1985). With this knowledge, Aloe was used by Heggers and other researchers in several burn environments, including high tension electricity burns, thermal (heat) burns, and frostbite.

Rabbits with frostbitten ears were treated with four different preparations, including Aloe. The control rabbits lost 100 percent of the frozen ear tissue by auto-amputation via tissue necrosis, while the Aloe-treated group retained 28.2 percent of such tissue (Heggers, 1985).

In a clinical setting, with 38 human patients who received a regimen of Aloe, penicillin, and aspirin, all patients healed. Only one patient experienced subsequent tissue loss, which was relatively minor (McCauley, 1982). "Robson and associates observed that tissue survival was enhanced (28.2% survival) when *Aloe vera* was used. In comparison, 17.5% survival occurred with topical methylprednisolone (Medrol) acetate" (McCauley, 1990, 68).

ALOE'S USE IN ELECTRICAL BURNS

Robson evaluated the use of Aloe in rats with induced high tension electrical burns. The control group rats auto-amputated (chewed) their legs off within 96 hours, showed increased levels of thromboxane, and lost a significant portion of their legs. With Aloe treatment, there was minimal increase in thromboxane, and significantly less leg loss (Robson, 1984).

ALOE'S USE IN HEAT BURNS

In studies of thermal (heat) burns, to determine the therapeutic value of Aloe, Heggers found the thermally injured tissue showed no evidence of injury three weeks post burn. More importantly, he found no thromboxane in the treated tissue. Says Heggers, "One may postulate, then, that the steriochemical configurations of the Aloe vera plant products ...[may have as] one of its most beneficial effects in preventing the synthesis of TxA2, a most potent and devastating vasoconstrictor" (Heggers, 1985, 71). In layman's terms, Aloe prevents the formation of a compound that constricts the movement of blood into the burn site, thereby denying tissue of oxygen, nourishment, and removal of toxic product waste, which causes more tissue to be destroyed.

In a study (Rodriquez-Bigas, 1988) of laboratory-induced burns in guinea pigs, four different regimens of treatment were followed: one group received Silvadine, a second group received salicylic acid cream (aspirin), a third group received an Aloe gel extract (Carrington Dermal Wound Gel), and the last received plain gauze dressings. The results showed an effective antimicrobial action for Silvadine and Aloe, but not for the salicylic acid cream. The time required to complete healing was 50 days for the control group (gauze dressings), and the only group that showed a significantly faster rate of healing was the Aloe-treated group, which healed in an average of 30 days. Bacterial counts were significantly decreased by the Silvadine and by the Aloe gel, but not by the salicylic acid. "As previously reported by Robson et al. the concentrated forms of Aloe appear to be highly bactericidal" (Rodriguez-Bigas, 1988, 388).

THE ANTIMICROBIAL EFFECT OF ALOE

The antimicrobial effect of Aloe has been shown by several investigators, as reported by Cera et. al., (1980). At a 20 percent concentration, the Aloe vera extract tested was ineffective. However, *in vitro* (in lab dishes) tests showed that freshly concentrated extracts of Aloe were very antimicrobial, and that concentrations as low as 60 percent had a remarkable bactericidal effect. An additional benefit is the simple fact that Aloe vera gel keeps second- and third-degree burns from drying out, which is one of the most painful aspects of burns (Ship, 1977).

A number of individual animal burn case studies have been reported where Aloe treatment was used. Two involved dogs with severe burns (Cera et. al., 1980). Both showed remarkable healing in relatively short periods of time. The authors noted that the Aloe treatment apparently prevented the sepsis (infection) generally associated with severe burns. Another involved a severely burned rhesus monkey that was not expected to survive (Cera et. al., 1982). The monkey recovered in excellent condition, and the clinician noted that Aloe demonstrated three major properties which are beneficial in thermal injury: anesthetic effect, broad spectrum antimicrobial effect, and anti-thromboxane effect.

THE USE OF ALOE ON RADIATION BURNS

The effect of Aloe on radiation burns was of particular

interest to dermatologists in the mid-1930s. At that time, so little was known about the nature of and treatment for such burns that the positive effects of Aloe seemed miraculous. In a dermatologists' panel discussion, several physicians had positive clinical results: "A patient had a radiation burn about the size of a 25 cent piece; it was not deep but was painful. After about three months of treatment with this [Aloe vera] ointment, the ulcer closed up completely." And," I have used it [Aloe vera extract] and the leaves of Aloe vera extensively on patients with roentgen ray dermatitis and have seen some good results..." (Combs & Scheer, 1936, 902).

In another reported case study, an individual with serious X-ray burns was treated with Aloe. The clinician reported that the results were "most encouraging" particularly since the open wound was more than two-years standing. The clinician made a particular point of making a compound from *fresh* leaves each day (Wright,1936).

Another reported case in which the physician had tried numerous therapies shows the frustration at that time, "Under my supervision the patient received at various times the following therapeutic measures: application of wet dressings of saline solution, boric acid, thioglycerol and cysteine hydrochloride; treatment with various bland and stimulating ointments: including bismuth subnitrate and neoarsphenamine; application of adhesive dressings, and superficial cauterization of the edges with the actual cautery. Little improvement was noted as a result of any of these measures." However, after seven months of Aloe gel treatments, the burn was healed (Loveman, 1937). No wonder the physician was thrilled with the Aloe treatment!

Interestingly, two clinicians during this early period

made sure they used *fresh* Aloe. Two Cincinnati physicians grew their own Aloe, then cut and applied the fresh leaves to patients immediately. Their main reason for doing so was the short supply of leaves and the expense to indigent patients (Fine & Brown, 1938). Little did they know that using fresh leaves preserved the most important medicinal characteristics of the plants.

Another researcher reported the use of Aloe on radiation burns of the mouth. Three months after radiation therapy a severe mouth radiation ulcer had developed. After applying fresh Aloe to the ulcer for some seven hours a day for eight weeks, pain relief was instant, and the ulcer healed (Mandeville, 1939).

Several researchers used more traditional animal studies to investigate Aloe's effect on radiation burns. Using rats, Rowe et. al. (1941) noted that Aloe was an effective treatment. "Sufficient data has been obtained to show that treatment with the pulp of the leaf definitely increases the rate of healing of such experimentally produced reactions [radiation burns]." Using rabbits, Lushbaugh and Hale (1953) noted that, "Epithelization in the areas treated with the [Aloe] ointment was macroscopically well advanced by the twentieth day but had not similarly advanced even by the thirtieth day in the untreated areas" (693). And, in a more recent study using mice, Strickland et. al. (1992) exposed the animals to sunlamps to induce UVB radiation. Measuring the skin's cellular immune response, the exposure reduced the response by 68 percent compared with the unradiated control group. Treatment with Aloe after the radiation completely preserved the skin's cellular immune response.

EXPLANATION OF CONFLICTING RESULTS

As has been pointed out in earlier chapters, not all studies showed positive results to Aloe treatment. However, it can be stated with considerable certainty that those studies showing no effect on burns were likely conducted with deficient Aloe, containing no active ingredients. Ashley et. al. (1957) found no positive effect on burns from Aloe, but it is not possible to determine whether they used *fresh* Aloe so as to be effective. If they used an ill-considered preparation, there would be no positive effect. Kaufman et. al. (1988) provides proof of the use of an ineffective Aloe in his study, noting in his report, "The AVG [Aloe Vera Gel] preparation consisted of a crude extract from the center of the leaves, kept at -19 degrees centigrade and thawed once a day before application" (157). With such a preparation and with such handling, no active ingredient would be left in the gel.

A STORY OF BURN HEALING USING ALOE VERA

As she sat at the table, turning over the hot chicken pot pie to remove it from its cooking tin, 8-year-old Mary wasn't careful enough. The steaming pie fell onto her legs just below her shorts. As she screamed in pain, her father remembered that his mother always kept an Aloe plant in the kitchen window above the stove for burns. He rushed next door where his neighbor had Aloe plants, and returned home with a big plant. As her parents applied the fresh Aloe to her tortured legs, Mary's pain began to subside. Within three hours, the purple coloring and blistering was gone. Mary put on her pajamas and went to bed (Magness, 1993). Pliny the Elder would not have been surprised.

6

ALOE VERA AS A TREATMENT IN DIABETES

Diabetes is a disease that afflicts more than 12 million Americans and is the third leading cause of death in the United States (Rector-Page, 1992). The greatest challenge to treating those suffering with diabetes is stabilizing blood sugar levels. However, what is not understood by many non-diabetics are the distressing foot problems associated with those abnormal sugar levels (Danhof, 1985).

Fourteen percent of all diabetic patients require hospitalization annually for foot problems related to diabetes (Rubinstein et al., 1983). The wounds in the feet of diabetic patients are five times more likely to become infected than wounds in the feet of non-diabetics (Davis et al., 1988). In contrast to other patients, diabetics have a paradoxical situation with which they have to cope. They complain of pain, cramps, and burning in their feet; yet, at the same time, diabetics are insensitive to painful stimuli much of the time, resulting in wounds of which they are unaware. Peripheral nerve damage resulting from the lack of blood circulation to the extremities causes nerve pathology–resulting in pain (Davis et al.,1988). However, when trauma occurs to the feet and there is a lack of normal sensation, the damaged tissue is often resistant to healing because of the poor supply of blood and the resultant poor vitality of the injured tissue, predisposing the wound to infection (Danhof, 1985).

FOOT CARE IN DIABETES

Three of the most critical manifestations of diabetes in foot care are: 1) the diminished ability of the foot to respond to fluid changes; 2) peripheral neuropathy (numbness or lack of response to painful stimuli); and 3) poor wound healing (Davis et al., 1988).

The diminished ability to respond to fluid changes is critical because swelling is a necessary step in wound healing. Osmotic pressure changes (which separates a solution in the body from a solvent) and peripheral dehydration cause fluid imbalances, making wound repair more difficult. Diabetics tend to show a decrease in the normal swelling that is necessary for optimal wound healing (Davis et al. 1988).

Peripheral neuropathy occurs in many diabetics because the nerves lose sensation. Not only does this cause numbness, tingling and burning, but it can also result in unperceived injuries.

Poor wound healing occurs in many diabetics. This deficiency could be attributed to many factors, but two are the poor performance of collagen connective tissue, and the premature aging of fibroblast tissue. Healthy fibroblast tissue begins the healing process.

THE USE OF ALOE VERA IN FOOT CARE IN DIABETES

Davis and a team of researchers (1988) conducted three separate tests to determine the effectiveness of Aloe vera in treating these three critical manifestations of diabetes in foot care. To determine the effectiveness of Aloe in treating wound healing specific to diabetes, experimental mice were injected with a substance causing the onset of diabetes. Forty-eight hours later, the diabetes was confirmed by testing blood sugar levels. Following the set-up, circular pieces of skin were removed from both the right and left sides of all mice involved. The first group of 12 mice was injected with 1 mg of fresh Aloe prepared daily. The second group of 12 mice were injected with 10 mg of the same Aloe. The third group of 12 received 100 mg of Aloe daily and the forth group received no treatment at all. The diabetic mice treated with Aloe for six days demonstrated increased rates of healing (when compared with the control group) on days four and seven.

Mice receiving more Aloe experienced more healing in a shorter amount of time, indicating a dose response curve. Those who received 1 mg and 10 mg of Aloe had the most outstanding percentage of wound reduction after six days. Those receiving 100 mg of Aloe demonstrated significant healing after only three days of treatment (Davis et al., 1988).

To address the issue of analgesia (the lack of pain while conscious), Davis and his research team (1988) used several groups of mice. One group of 12 diabetic mice was injected daily with 100 mg of Aloe for a week, while another group of diabetic mice was injected with a saline solution. Another group of non-diabetic mice was used to determine normal responses to pain, and was given no injections prior to the experiment. The mice were then placed on hotplates to determine their reaction to the pain. The diabetic mice who had been injected with Aloe vera were able to tolerate the painful stimuli a full three seconds longer than control, but did not demonstrate an obliteration of responsiveness to stimuli. Aloe activity appears to be different from most analgesic medication given to diabetes patients in that most diabetics respond strongly to analgesics and must have the dosage reduced by at least 50 percent of normal dosage so that they can tolerate it. However, the dosage of Aloe vera was *increased* to provide better results. Although Aloe seems to provide some pain relief, it does not dull stimuli important to diabetics.

THE USE OF ALOE VERA IN
THE TREATMENT OF EDEMA

A third study conducted by Davis and his research team (1988) addressed edema, swelling resulting from excessive accumulation of fluid in body tissue. For this experiment, diabetes was induced in three groups of rats. When pronounced diabetic, edema was induced in the three groups of rats. One group had received 10 mg of Aloe the day before, another group had received 100 mg of Aloe the day before, and a third group had received no treatment. The study indicated that the Aloe reduced edema in a dose response fashion. Five times more reduction in the edema was observed in the rats treated with Aloe vera than those receiving no treatment.

In another study addressing edema, gibberellin and Aloe were administered to adult male diabetic mice to determine the effect on blood levels. In the study, one group of diabetic mice received injections of gibberellin, a glycoside and growth hormone isolated in Aloe vera. A second group of mice received injections of Aloe vera, and a third group received a combination of Aloe and gibberellin, while a fourth group received no treatment. Gibberellin, Aloe, and the combination of the two all reduced edema. However, unlike steroids used to treat edema, the gibberellin and Aloe vera inhibited the inflammation without retarding the healing of wounds (Davis et al., 1989).

Studies have also been done using the isolated polysaccharides from Aloe vera to treat foot ulcers specifically related to diabetes. These studies revealed that when treated with botanically derived polysaccharides isolated from the Aloe vera plant, replication of fibroblasts was stimulated six times more than in those diabetics untreated (Danhof, 1985). It is postulated that the polysaccharides in Aloe vera may actually increase the circulation around the wound as is indicated by an increase in skin temperature (Danhof, 1985).

Dr. Danhof (1985) revealed a touching, and all too familiar story of a family with a diabetic family member. An 83-year-old diabetic woman had an ulcer on her left foot which had failed to respond to several treatment regimens over a period of several months. Doctors advised amputation before the infection spread. The family was not prepared to cope with such a drastic measure and began a search for a more conservative mode of treatment. In their search, the use of Aloe vera to treat the ulcerated foot was suggested. Within 14 weeks of cleansing and treating the wound with a polymannan, the wound was healed.

ALOE VERA'S EFFECT ON BLOOD SUGAR LEVELS

Further studies also addressed the area of blood sugar levels of diabetics. Hikino and his research team (1986) conducted one of the early studies using the polysaccharide components of Aloe vera to treat diabetic mice. The astonishing results indicated a significant hypoglycemic effect, much like that of insulin. In a similar study, it was demonstrated that when Aloe vera was ingested by diabetic patients, they experienced a significant decrease in their fasting blood sugar levels (Ghannam et al., 1986).

In mice studied for the effects of Aloe on insulin levels, it was determined that insulin levels were significantly increased four hours after the administration of Aloe vera in diabetic mice. In addition, their blood glucose levels remained lower for 24 hours following the administration of the Aloe vera (Beppu et al., 1991).

A study using one of the largest populations was conducted by Dr. Argawal (1985) in India in the 1980s. For his study, he used 5,000 patients, 3,167 of which were diabetic. After the administration of Aloe vera, he noted that fasting and postprandial (after eating) blood sugar levels in 2,990 of the patients dropped to normal. Ninety percent of the patients responded to Aloe as a treatment for the blood sugar level imbalances associated with diabetes (Argawal, 1984).

ALOE VERA AS A TREATMENT FOR EYE COMPLICATIONS RESULTING FROM DIABETES

Eye complications are another concern to those with diabetes. Argawal and his team of researchers noted that Aloe, when administered in combination with other anti-diabetic agents, was effective treating patients with eye complications. They also supported the adjuvant factor of Aloe vera by noting that

Aloe stimulates the reparative process and enhances the effects of other medications.

Diabetic patients are anxious to learn about more humane treatments for their disease and its complications. "Aloe vera has been proven to be an effective agent in the treatment of wounds, edema, and pain associated with diabetes" (Davis et al., 1988). These multiple discoveries of the benefits of Aloe vera in the treatment of diabetes could hold great potential for diabetics and their family members who use self-treatment or desire to prevent diabetic damage to vital organs.

7

TREATMENT OF CANCER:
THE BENEFITS OF ALOE AND
POLYMANNANS

Scientific data indicates that 30 percent of all Americans will contract some sort of cancer in their lifetime. Because 90 percent of all cancers are environmentally caused, they are also preventable. Of the environmental causes, diet and nutrition are by far the two most influential. America has 500 percent more incidences of breast and colon cancer when compared to the rest of the world, indicating a serious need to look at diet and nutrients (Rector-Page, 1992). Nutrients include all foods and plants with nutritional value or physical benefit. The importance of nutrients indicates a need to review the value of Aloe vera in the prevention and treatment of cancer.

THE ANTITUMOR EFFECTS OF ALOE VERA

Aloe vera has been studied extensively in regard to its effect on various cancers. It has been found to have antitumor activity (Imanishi, 1993). In a study done with human tumor cells in a lab setting, Aloe vera gel was found to be cytotoxic to tumor cells, meaning that it destroyed the tumor cells (Winters et al., 1981).

Tizard stated that "there is abundant evidence that some mannans and glycans are very potent anticancer agents" (Tizard, 1992, 286). He further explained that mannans (the active components in Aloe gel) induce macrophage activity, which causes the release of interleukin, the stimulation of bone marrow activity, and the inhibition of tumor growth (Tizard et al., 1989). As early as 1947, one study conducted by Diller indicated that polysaccharides showed antitumor activity when administered to mice with sarcoma (malignant tumor in the soft tissue).

INTERFERON TREATMENT

Interferon treatment in cancer patients is of great relevance when addressing the issue of the effectiveness of Aloe vera in treating cancer. Interferons are natural cellular proteins formed when cells are exposed to viruses or other foreign particles. The interferons protect cells from those viruses and foreign material. Our cells have multiple biochemical mechanisms to prevent virus and cancer-causing damage in our bodies. Interferon therapy, classified by oncologists as a biological therapy, is administered by injection or intravenously (Sherry, 1994). In human cells treated with interferon, there was a decrease in the production of tumors (Goldstein & Laszlo, 1986). It also has been shown to inhibit the growth of many types of tumors (Grander et al., 1990).

Edmonson and a team of researchers conducted a study in 1987 with 16 patients who had been diagnosed with incurable nonosseous sarcomas. All of them had undergone surgery, 10 had received radiation treatment, and 14 had received chemotherapy. All patients received interferon treatment. Although there was no regression of the cancer, the disease stabilized for more than eight weeks after they received the interferon treatment.

Interferon is reported to reduce tumors in 30 percent of patients treated with interferon therapy (Sherry, 1994). In cancer of the urinary tract, interferon treatment was effective in 15 percent of patients (Sherry, 1994). In the chronic stages of leukemia, interferon therapy is sometimes administered to control the white blood cell count (Sherry, 1994). Interferon therapy has proven to be "effective in the treatment of kidney cancer, melanoma, and lymphoma; this particular therapy has proven extremely effective in the treatment of a rare cancer known as hairy cell leukemia" (Sherry, 1994, p. 214).

Interferon therapy may become known as a fourth level treatment for cancer patients. It would be fourth after surgery, radiation treatment, and chemotherapy (Goldstein & Laszlo, 1986). As a fourth level treatment, it has been said to hold a bright future for the treatment of malignant diseases.

ALOE AND INTERFERON TREATMENT

One might wonder what the connection between interferon treatment in cancer patients and Aloe vera treatment in cancer patients might be. Lackovic et al., (1970), may have best summarized the connection with their finding that the mannans in polysaccharides stimulate natural interferon production in the body, Borecky et al., (1967) stated: "Mannans are well recognized as potent inducers of interferon activity." Another group of researchers stated: "Acemannan is taken up by macrophages in which it enhances release of interferon" (Kemp et al., 1990). In addition, "Manapol extract stimulates production of macrophages, interferon, lymphocytes, phagocytic white blood cells, prostaglandin E2 (PGE 2) and cytokines—all important components of immune response" (Schechter, 1994, 52). Therefore, it is critical to note that not only does the mannan in Aloe vera have antitumor activity in and of itself, but it also stimulates interferon which has antitumor activity. Acemannan also stimulates T-Cell activity which may contribute to reduction in tumors (Womble & Helderman, 1988).

POLYMANNANS AND CANCER TREATMENT

The polymannans have been researched fairly thoroughly using dogs and cats as subjects. In one study, 43 animals, 32 dogs and 11 cats, ranging from ages three to seventeen years old, and all with malignant tumors, were used. All the animals had been classified in one or more of the three following ways: there was no effective conventional treatment for their malignancies; they had failed to respond to conventional treatments; or the disease was too advanced for clinical treatment. All animals were treated with acemannan at least every three weeks for at least five treatments. Seven of the animals died after only one treatment, indicating that they were really too progressed in their disease to participate in the study. Thirteen showed no significant clinical response. One demonstrated no response after a full course of therapy. Twelve of the animals, eight dogs and four cats, demonstrated obvious clinical improvement, based on tumor shrinkage, tumor necroses (the disappearing of the tumor), or an unexpectedly long survival. Many of the soft sarcomas increased in size due to localized increased vascular permeability, which is a positive prognostic sign. Six of the animals had tumors that had been encapsulated, rendering previously inoperable tumors operable. It is postulated that the macrophage activation caused by the polymannans may contribute to encapsulation in the area of tumors. The study found fibrosarcomas to be especially amenable to the therapy (Harris et al., 1991).

Another study also investigated the effectiveness of B-(1,4)-linked mannan treatment with fibrosarcoma. Fibrosarcomas are among the most frequently occurring tumors in dogs. The study employed four dogs and six cats diagnosed with the disease. All the animals received from three to twelve injections of acemannan. Tumor shrinkage was noted in two animals. Eight of the animals exhibited swelling in the tumor which has been noted as a positive prognostic sign, indicating gross tumor necrosis (death of the tumor tissue). Four of the animals required no further treatment after the acemannan injections. In six of the animals, the residual tumor was removed surgically. Eighteen months following the study, three of the animals remained free of tumors. An additional animal was tumor free when it died due to unrelated causes five months later. Seven of the animals that still had tumors demonstrated tumor necrosis. Encapsulation of the tumor was seen in two animals. It was concluded that "acemannan has a positive therapeutic effect on fibrosarcomas of dogs and cats; thus it should be a safe and useful adjunct to the treatment of fibrosarcoma" (King & Pierce, 1992, 13).

In another study, female mice were induced with sarcoma cells. Usually this strain of mice dies within 20 to 46 days of the onset of sarcoma. In this study, it was shown that the B-(1,4)-linked mannan treatment increased survival. When the treatment was reduced, the survival time also was reduced proportionately. With the treatment, tumor regression happened 12 to 15 days from the time of treatment. There was a variety in the effectiveness of tumor reduction. Some of the mice demonstrated moderate tumor reduction, some experienced complete resorption of the tumor.

The survival rate of the mice receiving the treatment was 35 to 40 percent. This may seem like a low survival rate, but it is quite significant when realizing that of the mice receiving no treatment, 100 percent died. The results of this study indicate that "acemannan stimulates macrophage synthesis of immunologically stimulatory monokines and causes growth regression of a murine solid tumor...a poorly differentiated sarcoma" (Peng et al., 1991, 86).

In a discussion regarding the same study, Tizard (1992, 287) explained some of the above results. He stated that "animals treated intraperitoneally with acemannan at the time of sarcoma cell implantation synthesize a cytotoxic factor(s) initiating necrosis and regression of the rapidly growing subcutaneous sarcomas." He further explained that the acemannan also enhances other functions of the macrophage, such as phagocytosis (the surrounding, engulfing and disposing of cell debris) and cytotoxicity (removal of toxins that damage or destroy tissue cells) (Tizard, 1992).

POLYMANNANS AND LEUKEMIA

A group of researchers conducted a study using cats with feline leukemia. Normally, 40 percent of cats are dead within four weeks of the onset of these clinical symptoms, and 70 percent are dead eight weeks after onset, rendering it an excellent clinical disease for studying the effectiveness of treatment with B-(1,4)-linked mannans. Of the 44 cats employed in the study, 29 were still alive at the end of the study, a 71 percent survival rate when treated with acemannan. The administration of acemannan was conducted for six weeks. Eight weeks after the study, 21 owners stated that their cats were still alive and functioning normally. They had "returned to their normal state of activity and were happy, healthy pets" (Sheets et al., 1991, 43). The results indicated that "the significant improvement in viability as well as the overall health of the treated cats suggests that acemannan is an effective treatment of feline leukemia virus-infected cats" (Sheets et al., 1991, 45). Tizard (1991, 1484) stated that the results of this study "are encouraging, because they provide, for the first time, a possible mode of treatment for this disease." Leukemia is diagnosed in 28,000 people annually in the United States, and is the most common childhood cancer (Sherry, 1994). Because it is inoperable, and there have previously been few, if any, successful treatment regimens, the results of the studies using the polymannans hold promise for further study and possible future treatment of leukemia in humans.

As a result of these, and other studies, "Manapol® extract has received conditional approval from the U.S. Department of Agriculture (USDA) as an aid in the treatment of canine and feline fibrosarcoma—cancer in underlying tissue such as muscle, bone, and connective tissue" (Schechter, 1994, 52). As these studies progress, perhaps they will be approved for trials in humans.

THE EFFECTIVENESS OF POLYMANNANS IN THE TREATMENT OF OTHER CANCERS

Cancer of the liver has also been studied in regard to the effectiveness of treatment with B-(1,4)-linked mannans. Three groups of male rats were used to conduct one study. One group of 20 rats received a 30 percent Aloe vera diet for eight days prior to exposure to carcinogens. A second group of 20 rats received no treatment prior to exposure to carcinogens. A third group of five rats received no exposure to carcinogens. It was noted that the first group, supplemented with an Aloe vera diet experienced some protection from the carcinogens, indicating that the Aloe acted as a preventive agent to hepatotoxins, inhibiting hepatocarcinogenesis (liver cancer) (Tsuda et al., 1993].

In regard to various other cancers, Dr. Vorontsov found Aloe treatment helpful in the following conditions: cancer of the esophagus, stomach, intestines, mammary gland, skin, mucosa of mouth and lips, and female genitalia in stages III to IV. He noted that in female genitalia tumors, Aloe treatment resulted in decreased discharges and that secondary inflammatory complications abated. In general, he noted that treatment with Aloe helped inhibit tumor growth and improved the patient's general physical condition (Aryayew et al.).

THE ADJUVANT ACTIVITY OF B-(1,4)-LINKED MANNANS

Certainly not to be overlooked is the adjuvant activity of the B-(1,4)-linked mannans (Chinnah et al., 1992). Although the mannans hold promise in some cancer treatments in their own right, they also combine well with chemotherapy by boosting its performance and by decreasing its toxicity to bone marrow, liver and kidneys (McDaniel, 1994).

THE STORY OF A BRAVE SOLDIER

This brings the touching story of the fight of a brave

little soldier, my dear friend, Zita, to my mind. After being diagnosed with cancer, her health degenerated very quickly. She was hospitalized in a facility connected with a medical university. Although she never claimed to be a physician or scientist, Zita believed in using "what the good Lord created to treat illness." She requested that the physicians use acemannan adjunctively with her treatment. However, due to regulatory environment in force on new drug use in the United States, they denied her request. Zita obtained acemannan through veterinary channels where it has been effective for the treatment of cancer since 1989, and injected it herself. Although the treatment came late in her disease, her T-cell count, general energy, and state of well being did improve with the acemannan injections, despite her far advanced cancer status. Zita, a dear friend, mom, sister, aunt, and grandmother will be missed by all who knew her. However, her legend and her courage live on in all of us who knew her.

8

USES OF ALOE IN DIGESTIVE DISORDERS

The application of Aloe to digestive disorders is the oldest recorded use of the plant. From the earliest times, Aloe was a known laxative. For centuries, this use was the only use mentioned. Today, however, Aloe has shown that it has properties useful to other aspects of digestion and the digestive tract. Murray (1994, 54) states that, "Andrew Weil, M.D., of the University of Arizona at Tucson, reported that Aloe vera is beneficial in the treatment of various gastrointestinal complaints." Until recently, no distinction had been made between phytochemicals made in the cuticle (covering) of the leaf and those made in the central gel. The bitter flavor of whole leaf products is from chemicals in the outer part of the leaf and is responsible for its laxative effect. Manapol® is free of this toxic substance from the cuticle.

THE USE OF ALOE VERA
IN TREATING PEPTIC ULCERS

Research has been done on Aloe as a treatment for peptic ulcers. Grindlay and Reynolds (1986) reported on a study (done in 1963) of 12 patients with confirmed peptic ulcers (duodenal lesions). The patients were given an emulsion of Aloe vera, and the investigators claimed the ulcers were completely cured by the treatments, reporting that the ulcers had not reappeared even after a year's time. This is unusual, stated the researchers, because such "unmistakable lesions are accompanied by exacerbations of distress once and more often twice a year under any form of medical treatment, but no such episodes were experienced in this series of cases" (Grindlay and Reynolds, 1986, 130). X-rays showed complete healing. The researchers attributed the effect of the Aloe to inhibition of hydrochloric acid secretion and a general detoxifying effect.

ALOE AS A PREVENTION FOR ULCERS

Polymannans were found to be effective as an ulceroprotective in rats that had induced ulcers (McAnalley, 1989). The rats were given a single dose of Aloe extract orally two hours before the ulcerative material was given. Upon examination of the rats' stomachs, the treatment was found to be protective. Administration of the Aloe concurrently with the ulcerative material was not effective. When Aloe was given for several days prior to inducement of ulcers, the protective mechanism worked. Moreover, "Aloe extract was also effective when injected intraperitoneally, even when given concurrently with reserpine (the ulcerative material). This result suggested that the therapeutic action was at least partially systemic, rather than simply local in nature, and that a therapeutic blood concentration was attained more rapidly after parenteral administration" (McAnalley, 1989, 6015).

ALOE AS A DIGESTIVE AID

Aloe has demonstrated an ability to increase bile production, which in some cases is needed to aid digestion. Hazelton's study (1942) showed that release of bile was increased in dogs given Aloe. "The intravenous injection of extract of Aloe was followed by a 42 percent increase in the average bile production within the experimental interval of four 30-minute periods. In the three experiments which were prolonged for three or four 30-minute periods beyond the usual experimental interval, the rate of biliary flow continued to increase or remained at a high level. Inclusion of these results brings the average increase over the control value to 58 percent..." (Hazelton, 1942, 55).

ALOE AND COLON HEALTH

Bland (1985) studied the digestive effects of Aloe on 10 healthy humans. The subjects supplemented their diets with an Aloe vera juice preparation, but otherwise kept their normal eating habits. Several measurements of digestive health were taken. "The most marked objective difference between the pre-Aloe and post-Aloe supplementation periods in the various subjects was the decrease in stool specific gravity indicating a greater water-holding characteristic of the stool and improved gastrointestinal motility with reduced bowel transit time. This would indicate that the Aloe vera supplementation had a tonic effect on the intestinal tract. This mild tonic effect was not accompanied by any diarrhea and, therefore, would not be considered operating as a true laxative" (Bland, 1985, 137).

The dietary supplementation also altered the bacterial characteristics of the colon. "Those subjects that had heavy overgrowth of fecal bacteria and some yeast infection, were found to have improved fecal colonization and decreased yeast after the Aloe vera juice supplementation" (Bland, 1985, 137). Protein digestion efficiency was increased, and "the indication that dietary protein is better absorbed and less available for putrification may also indicate why some individuals have in the past found Aloe vera to be helpful in the management of various food allergic symptoms or arthritis-like pain" (137).

ALOE AS A TREATMENT FOR ULCERATIVE COLITIS

One of the most important uses for Aloe in digestive health may be in the treatment of ulcerative colitis. McDaniel (1995) commented on the use of a B-(1,4)-linked mannan in the treatment of this debilitating disease, "[In a 1986] FDA sanctioned clinical pilot study for treating ulcerative colitis and Crohn's disease using a relatively crude freeze-dried Aloe product formulated in capsules that he states was inferior in its bioactivity to the current oral polymannan known as Manapol®. The results were very encouraging for this poorly managed disease for which there is no known cause, cure, or good treatment. In 1993-94, a six-center clinical study for treatment of colitis with oral acemannan was conducted with Vanderbilt Medical Center Gastroenterology Department as the primary investigator site. The report on these colitis patients' response to oral acemannan to the FDA has provided the basis to start a Phase II clinical study projected to start in 1995. There is no question of the high degree of effectiveness oral polymannans will have in this difficult disease. Hundreds of these types of patients have used the polymannans available as a nutritional supplement Manapol and have had relief of signs and symptoms in a few days. These were patients unresponsive to all currently used toxic drugs," McDaniel stated in an interview.

ALOE AS A LAXATIVE

The oldest known use for Aloe as a plant medication was as a laxative. As noted in an earlier chapter, the active compound for this laxative effect is Aloin, and its effectiveness is not seriously questioned in the medical community. Although constipation can be a problem for persons of any age, it is a particularly serious medical problem in the elderly.

Several studies have confirmed Aloe's effectiveness as a laxative. Chapman & Pittelli (1974) studied a then-common commercial laxative which contained two active ingredients, phenolphthalein and Aloin. The double-blind, crossover comparison study was to determine the effect of each of the components as compared with the combination. The study showed that both active ingredients worked, but that the combination was more effective than either separately. The number of subjects reporting adverse experiences did not vary greatly between the compounds taken. None of the adverse experiences were reported to be more serious than "mild."

In a similar study of combination laxatives (Odes & Madar, 1991), Aloe was combined with celandin, and psyllium. Thirty-five men and women received the compound or a placebo in a 28-day, double-blind trial. "Symptoms in the last two weeks of the treatment period were compared to those in the 14-day pretrial basal period. In the celandin, Aloe vera and psyllium group, bowel movements became more frequent, the stools were softer, and laxative dependence was reduced. In the placebo group, all these parameters were unchanged. Abdominal pain was not reduced in either group. The results show that the preparation is an effective laxative in the treatment of constipation" (Odes, 1991, 65).

9

ADVANCES IN TREATING AIDS: THE PROMISE OF ALOE

Every 15 seconds, someone new contracts the dreaded virus, AIDS (acquired immunodeficiency syndrome) (Greene, 1993). Although it has been more than 15 years since the virus was first identified and brought to public awareness, there is still no cure, effective treatment, or vaccine. The virus is one of the principle threats to human life worldwide (Greene, 1993). The Global AIDS Policy Coalition projects that by the year 2000, there will be 40-110 million people infected with the disease, which is 2 percent of the world's population.

Previously, many people were naive regarding the virus, assuming that it only affected the homosexual community. However, the majority of new cases of the virus are now from heterosexual contact (Greene, 1993). Women account for 40 percent of AIDS cases, and another 10 percent are children born to mothers infected with the virus (Greene, 1993). For these many reasons, the human immunodeficiency virus (HIV) and the acquired immunodeficiency syndrome

(AIDS) are the most intensively studied viruses in our history.

HOW THE VIRUS ATTACKS THE BODY

The syndrome is a complex set of events that occurs once the body is exposed to the virus. Initially, the body produces a massive immune defense to the virus. During this defensive move, Beta cells produce antibodies that neutralize the virus. Killer T-cells then multiply en mass in order to destroy all those cells that have been infected with the virus. As a result, the immune system seems to successfully fight off the virus in its early phase.

A person who has contracted the disease initially experiences flu-like symptoms which dissipate in a short period of time. The flu-like symptoms concur with the initial defense phase. When it seems the virus is being fought off successfully, the flu-like symptoms disappear, and the virus actually remains low grade, multiplying at a slow but steady pace for a number of years.

By the time the virus is detectable in the blood, sometimes years later, the infection is usually out of control Some researchers believe that the virus is actively growing in the lymph nodes. After years of inflicting damage to the immune system, opportunistic malignancies and infections begin to occur in the body. This is the most common time when the actual diagnosis is made.

At this point, however, the illness is being caused by the human immunodeficiency virus. Most researchers believe that HIV is the primary cause of AIDS, and that even those who do not develop AIDS experience profound immune dysfunction over time (Greene, 1993).

Presently (1995), the major treatment for HIV and AIDS is supportive. Patients are placed on nutritional programs to provide optimal health, they are placed on appropriate exercise programs, and they receive medical treatment for whatever infections are present.

ALOE VERA IS CONSIDERED
AS A TREATMENT FOR AIDS

Aloe vera has long been known for its unique treatment capabilities or its remedial properties for skin and bowel illnesses. This limited range of effectiveness and use only as a folk medicine is why some believed that studying Aloe as a treatment for AIDS was ludicrous.

In the 1989 Dallas Morbidity Report, it was stated that some groups were suggesting the use of Aloe vera juice to treat AIDS, but labeled such claims about Aloe as "fraud" (Green, 1989). However, in that same year, 1989, the *Times Picayune* in New Orleans, LA., made a very different statement: "A substance in the Aloe plant shows preliminary signs of boosting AIDS patients' immune systems and blocking the human immunodeficiency virus' spread without toxic effects."

The road to such tests and results has been long and hard, not only because of the process required by the Food and Drug Administration (FDA), but because of overcoming "fraud" statements and many opinions like the first one mentioned above.

FDA's PROTOCOL FOR APPROVING NEW DRUGS

The Congressional Office of Technology Assessment conducted a study in 1993 to determine the costs for pharmaceutical companies to follow the FDA's protocol for making drugs available to the public through physician prescription. The cost is about $359 million and is averaged over 12 years. Only one in 5,000 experimental drugs ever makes it to the stage of human testing after being tested in labs and with animals. When some trials have been successful, it can sometimes be administered to critically ill patients on "compassionate grounds."

In an article published in the *Fort Worth Star-Telegram* (Finn, 1994), the director of the AIDS Coordinating Council of Tarrant County expressed the frustration of patients suffering with the virus when drugs with new promise are reported on, and patients cannot obtain the drugs. "You had drugs that looked good in the lab and you couldn't get them. Your survival rate with AIDS is zero. So the drug kills you. What have you lost? It might work. There was a lot of anger out there." Finally, successful pilot trials in Dallas (3), Belgium (1), and Canada (1) on human subjects have made the nutritional supplement sources of polymannans derived from the Aloe plant more available.

ANTIVIRAL THERAPY USING POLYMANNANS

General antiviral therapy has been studied for decades. The rationale for AIDS therapy is that if an individual is able to maintain a state in which HIV replication is suppressed, they can remain free from the opportunistic infections which many times lead to death. In the meantime, the immune system, if not totally damaged, can regenerate healthy CD4 cells, and the lymphocyte numbers may return to normal, or near normal (Balzarini & Broder., 1988).

The polymannans have been shown to be antiviral. It appears that they enhance the immune system by increasing the generation of and improving the function of cytotoxic T-cells which are generated to combat virally infected cells (Womble & Helderman, 1992). In addition, it has been repeatedly demonstrated that antiviral cytokines produced by leukocytes can be induced by polymannans.

THE USE OF POLYMANNANS
TO TREAT AIDS AND HIV

Studies have resulted in powerful statements regarding the use of polymannans as antiviral agents. These quotes have been taken directly from researchers working in laboratory settings with this substance: "Acemannan holds an important promise as a clinically useful antiviral agent" (Womble & Helderman, 1992, 76); "There is now mounting evidence that acemannan may be an agent capable of delimiting infections to DNA and retro-viruses that cause significant disease in animal and man" (Womble & Helderman, 1988, 972); "Acemannan's capacity to inhibit viral replication, combined with its immunostimulatory capabilities, indicates that acemannan may also be useful in the treatment of human immunodeficiency virus (HIV), which causes acquired immunodeficiency syndrome (AIDS)" (Investigator Brochure, 1992, 1); "They [mannans] are potent immunostimulants with significant activity against infectious diseases and tumors" (Tizard et al., 1989).

The studies to determine the effectiveness of polymannans, derived from Aloe, in treating HIV and AIDS have been going on since the 1980s, with much of the research being conducted in the Dallas, Texas area. "For AIDS/HIV, the most systematic studies are being done by advocates of Carrisyn[®], a chemical found in Aloe vera and now being moved through the FDA approval process by Carrington Laboratories in Dallas, Texas" (James, 1989, 388).

USING POLYMANNANS TO TREAT HIV SYNERGISTICALLY

There have been other studies that have supported the use of mannans in the treatment of HIV. The polymannans have been shown to enhance and sustain the magnitude of immune response when used to treat Newcastle disease. This is a virus which is very similar to HIV, indicating that it may be effective in enhancing the immune system's response to HIV (Chinnah et al., 1992).

One of the greatest uses of polymannans is in synergy

with other drugs. It has been shown that polymannans have direct antiviral properties against HIV, that they are non-cytotoxic at high concentrations, and that they work synergistically with AZT, the primary medication for treatment of AIDS (Kahlon et al., September 1991).

In order for drugs to be considered for combination therapy with other drugs in the treatment of HIV, they must: act synergistically to inhibit HIV replication; not have the same toxicity as the first medication; prevent or delay the development of the virus; be able to suppress the immunosuppressive effect of HIV to assist in preventing opportunistic infections; counteract toxicity; have different tissue distributions; have different cell tropisms; and have antiviral and immuno-enhancing properties (Yarchoan et al., 1990). The polymannans appear to fit these criterion.

AZT AND ALOE IN THE TREATMENT OF AIDS

Azidothymidine (AZT) is currently the only approved drug for the treatment of AIDS. However, it has many cytotoxic effects, such as granuloctyopenia (blood disorders), anemia, headaches, myalgia, anorexia, diarrhea, nausea, vomiting, dizziness, insomnia, taste perversion, paresthesia (numbness and tingling, mostly in the extremities), and somnolence (drowsiness) (Physicians Desk Reference, 1994). This toxicity makes the long term use of AZT and other antiviral treatments such as ddC, ddI, and interferon alone nearly impossible (Clumeck & Hermans, 1988). Many researchers believe that the amount of AZT administered will be reduced and synergistic treatment with other more benign antiviral agents will increase (Kahlon et al., September 1991). This makes studies regarding the synergism between AZT and acemannan very attractive.

Studies indicate that acemannan inhibits viral replication, increases the viability of infected cells, suppresses the formation of virus-induced syncytium cells (abnormally connected cells), and causes a reduction in virus load (Kemp et al.; Kahlon et al., September, 1991). In addition, studies have indicated that acemannan acts synergistically with AZT against HIV-1 and with ACY against herpes to inhibit HIV in lab culture studies (Kahlon et al., September 1991, December 1991). Acemannan has also been shown to stimulate the secretion of cytokines (which control the healing pathway) and the secretion of monocytes (Marshall et al., 1993). All of these properties make it an excellent candidate for synergistic use. "While acemannan alone might not be considered potent enough for antiviral therapy, it probably is for combination therapy, wherein compounds are selected for their ability to act synergistically to reduce toxicity and to enhance anti-viral efficacy" (Kahlon et al., September 1991, 134).

This synergism is of critical importance because of its potential in protecting mankind from a virus that could spread rampantly, producing countless deaths, unless a vaccine or effective treatment is found. "This finding in itself is important, but in terms of therapeutic value, if acemannan could be similarly shown to act synergistically with other antivirals and inhibit replication of viruses that cause extensive morbidity for the population as a whole, thus its potential therapeutic value could well be dramatically enhanced" (Kahlon et al., December 1991, 219).

STUDIES USING ACEMANNAN TO TREAT AIDS IN HUMANS

THE PILOT STUDY
The exploratory pilot study done for treating humans with acemannan used sixteen patients. The patients received 1,000 mg of acemannan daily for three months. Their symptoms were significantly reduced. The evaluation was done by Walter Reed Clinical Classification before the study and after treatment. All fever and night sweats were eliminated, there was improvement in or elimination of opportunistic infections and diarrhea, the HIV positive cells in culture were eliminated or reduced, and HIV core antigen levels dropped (McDaniel et al., 1987). In addition, 15 of the 16 had an increase in red cell mass. There were no toxic effects noted. Three months later, six of the 16 patients with very advanced AIDS showed 20 percent improvement in symptoms. Those who were less seriously ill showed an improvement of 71 percent.

THE PREDICTIVE PILOT STUDY
In 1986, patients were treated with acemannan for HIV or AIDS for a predictive pilot study. After the study was completed, the patients were allowed to continue their acemannan treatment on a gratis basis. The four patients who opted to continue their treatment were alive more than 84 months (seven years) after the study was completed. They had reported no serious opportunistic infections, and had no hospitalizations. Their CD4+ lymphocyte counts remained

stable and normal (or slightly below normal). Some of their lymphocyte counts rose to three times the level prior to acemannan treatment. They gained weight and were able to remain or become gainfully employed (McDaniel et al., 1994).

THE BELGIAN PILOT STUDY

One of the early pilot studies done on humans regarding the effectiveness of polymannans was conducted in Belgium. In the Belgian study, asymptomatic HIV and ARC (Aids Related Complex) infected patients were recruited for a double-blind, placebo-controlled study. The 47 patients, 10 females and 37 males, age 23 to 67 years old, were treated orally for 24 weeks.

One group received 800 mg of acemannan and a placebo daily. A second group received only a placebo. The third group received 800 mg of acemannan and AZT daily. The final group received AZT and a placebo daily (Weerts et al., 1990). The AZT group experienced an increase in incidence of adverse events or side effects. There was no difference in the incidence of adverse events in the acemannan and placebo groups. There were no safety concerns with the use of acemannan. Acemannan and AZT combination therapy resulted in elevated CD4+ cell counts, which was maintained for at least six months following the study. The group treated with AZT alone had some increase in CD4+ cell counts, but the increases were transient, not stable. The study demonstrated that acemannan improved the symptoms of ARC. Those treated with acemannan had a life expectancy nine to ten months longer than patients not treated with acemannan (Weerts et al., 1990).

CONFIRMATORY PILOT STUDY

In a 1987 confirmatory pilot study, 15 HIV-1 patients who received acemannan showed a 69 percent improvement in the first 90 days of treatment. They experienced a reduction in the severity and incidence of opportunistic infections, while the infections were eliminated all together in some cases. They experienced weight gains and returned to normal physical activity (McDaniel et al., 1994).

THE CANADIAN STUDY

In January of 1991, it was announced in the *Network Update* that studies evaluating the combination treatment of AZT and acemannan would begin in Vancouver and Calgary, Canada. Sixty volunteers, already being treated with AZT, would be treated by adding acemannan to their current treatment for one year. Patients with advanced HIV were used for the double-blind, placebo-controlled study, which was conducted under the auspices of the Canadian HIV Clinical Trials Network. The objective was to determine the effectiveness of acemannan on CD4+ decline, being used as a primary indicator of HIV disease progression. Those patients who received acemannan and AZT in combination therapy showed significant stabilization of CD4+ counts between weeks 16 and 48. "The study confirmed that acemannan is a safe medication" (News Release, 1992).

FELINE IMMUNODEFICIENCY VIRUS

Many studies have been conducted with cats to

determine the effects of B-(1,4)-linked mannans on feline immunodeficiency virus (FIV), which is similar to HIV in humans (Pedersen et al., 1991). Veterinarians call this disease "feline AIDS," and it is a model used in AIDS research. The feline immunodeficiency virus is spread primarily through bites from infected animals.

There are five stages in the progression of the disease. Stage one is similar to the onset of HIV in that it is characterized by flu-like symptoms which normally subside in a few weeks. Stage two is asymptomatic as the CD4+ cells gradually but progressively decrease. One third or more of infected cats are taken to the veterinarian for treatment in stage three. In this stage, there is normally recurrent fever, lymph node disorders, and some anorexia. In stage four, the chronic secondary infections begin, characterized by weight loss and blood disorders. Half of these animals have symptoms similar to ARC or AIDS in humans. In stage five, chronic infections increase in severity until the cat dies, usually within one to six months (Pedersen et al., 1991; Yates et al., 1992).

One study of cats infected with FIV was conducted with 49 cats in stages three to five. Twenty-three had severe lymphopenia (a decreased number of lymphocytes in the peripheral circulation, like AIDS). For treatment, the cats were divided into three groups. Group one had acemannan administered intravenously once weekly, while group two had acemannan administered subcutaneously (by injection just beneath the skin) weekly. A third group received acemannan orally on a daily basis.

Lab analyses were done at the beginning of the study,

at week six and at week 12. These analyses indicated no significant differences in the effectiveness of the acemannan administered through the three different routes. However, all the cats experienced significant increases in their lymphocyte counts, with significant reduction in neutrophil counts. (Neutrophil counts normally rise when there is acute infection present).

The survival rate for all three groups was 75 percent. Thirty six of the 49 animals used for the study were still alive 19 months after the study. "These results suggest that acemannan therapy may be of significant benefit in FIV-infected cats exhibiting clinical signs of disease" (Yates et al., 1992, 177). In addition, there were no adverse side effects in any of the animals treated with acemannan (Yates et al., 1992).

HOPE FOR HIV+ AND AIDS PATIENTS

Although these results are incredibly hopeful, there are warnings about labeling acemannan as a cure-all for AIDS or HIV infected patients. "Acemannan is not considered a possible 'cure' for AIDS. Rather, it would arrest the progression of the disease, enabling the patient to live out a more or less normal lifespan when used in conjunction with AZT, the most widely used medication for AIDS" (Pullin, 1994). However, the results of the studies reviewed in this chapter make it difficult not to feel inspired by results obtained to date. Dr. Faith Strickland of M.D. Anderson Hospital in Houston, Texas, stated that she had great hope about the use of Aloe in treating the viruses: "Aloe vera can not only stop the damage done to the immune system, but can actually restore it to full working order" (Pullin, 1994).

For AIDS and HIV infected patients and their loved ones, such results hold not only hope for future advances in treatment, but hope for life!

10

THE USE OF ALOE VERA IN SKIN PRODUCTS AND COSMETICS

There seems to be a "return to Mother Nature" in the cosmetic industry. "There is a tendency in today's pharmaceutical cosmetic markets to move away from synthetic ingredients and return to natural botanicals whenever possible. Aloe vera is certainly one of the more complex and widely recognized natural botanicals yet discovered" (Bowles, 1992, 22).

Legends say that Queen Nefertiti and Cleopatra, known for their striking beauty, both bathed in Aloe vera. Although we don't know whether or not the legend is factual, we do know that "Aloe vera's ingredients can help moisturize the skin, help regenerate dead skin, and tighten facial tissue. The compounds within the gel can also help eliminate acne, blackheads, and liver spots" (Taylor-Donald).

Many cosmetic companies attempt to increase the

sales of their products by claiming that they contain Aloe vera. Although these claims might be true, it is important to realize that the use of products with improperly processed Aloe vera might be the same even if the Aloe vera were present. Many of these products that claim to have Aloe in them have other toxic ingredients, making the presence or absence of Aloe irrelevant. Some of these toxins should be avoided.

To address the issue regarding products claiming to contain Aloe, Drs. Danhof and McAnalley conducted some studies to determine the actual content and effectiveness of various products. The results indicated that some products contained stabilized Aloe vera, some contained little or no Aloe vera, and some contained cytotoxic preservatives. They warned that "stabilized Aloe vera that is used on skin or in products intended for use on skin should be tested to show that its beneficial effects have been preserved" (Danhof & McAnalley, 1983, 110).

ALOE VERA AND COLLAGEN

Because of the age-old belief that Aloe is helpful to the skin, many of us are more drawn to products that claim they contain Aloe vera. One study evaluated the benefit of Aloe vera to the collagen, in our skin, which determines how flexible and supple our skin is. Aging is associated with the loss of collagen which results in wrinkling and creasing of the skin. The study used the skin of guinea pigs, applying Aloe vera daily for one and a half to four months. A second group received another topical application with no Aloe vera in it. The results demonstrated an increase in the collagen in the skin of the guinea pigs being treated with Aloe vera (Stachow et al., 1984).

ALOE VERA AND AGING SPOTS

Another study was done to determine the effectiveness of Aloe vera on "aging" or "liver" spots. These spots result from melanocytes, which when combined with amino acid, synthesize the brown skin pigment called melanin. Studies indicate that Aloe contains a tyrosinase, which can stop the formation of melanin (Ando et al., 1977). Another study indicated that in cosmetic creams with properly processed Aloe vera, the characteristics of aging skin were improved by rehydrating the skin and giving it "restorative" effects (Danhof, Aloe in Cosmetics).

ALOE VERA AS A MOISTURIZER

Although there are numerous miraculous cosmetic claims about the benefits of Aloe vera, "only those relating to the emollient moisturizing and healing properties of the gel seem to be documented in reputable scientific journals"

(Leung, 1978, 67). It is commonly accepted that these properties in Aloe vera gel are due to the polysaccharides present, more specifically the glucomannans (Leung, 1978).

The mannans in Aloe vera are effective in moisturizing the skin because of their ability to penetrate the skin, supplying moisture directly to the tissue. In addition, the gel forms a protective barrier to the skin, preventing loss of moisture from evaporation (Waller, 1992).

Aloe vera is effective in skin care because it is able to penetrate all three layers of the skin: the epidermis, dermis and hypodermis. It also has the ability to flush the bacteria and oil out that can clog our pores. Then the natural nutrients in fresh Aloe can stimulate growth of healthy new cells (Cassidy).

ALOE VERA AS A TREATMENT FOR EXPOSURE TO ELEMENTS

Aloe is also widely used in skin conditions resulting from exposure to the elements. It is excellent for treating sunburn, wind-chapped hands and faces, and chapped lips. Aloe is effective, because, in addition to the moisturizing ability of Aloe mentioned above, it is also known to be a natural pain reliever when applied topically, naturally soothing areas of tender skin (Cassidy).

ALOE VERA AND HAIR CARE

Another interesting cosmetic use of Aloe vera is in the area of hair care and baldness. I have heard it stated by several women that "90 percent of their self esteem was in their hair." This message began being imparted from childhood when stories like Rapunzel and Goldilocks were told. However, the quest for lustrous hair is nothing new. Pliny the Elder, back in 35 AD suggested using Aloe in a mixture with astringent wine to prevent hair from "falling off the head." In the Philippines, Aloe is also mixed with wine to treat baldness (Danhof, 1991,1992). When used for hair care, Aloe opens pores, cleanses the scalp, brings impurities to the surface, and restores healthy tissue to the scalp. Because it can penetrate the hair shaft, it is a very good agent for conditioning.

Many of us look for keratin, a natural substance known to promote healthy hair, when buying hair care products. Aloe vera is very similar to keratin in its chemical composition, helping to revitalize hair and protecting it from breakage (Cassidy).

Aloe vera for cosmetic use is not limited to the United States. European countries are also incorporating Aloe vera into their cosmetic products more and more. Many European cosmetic companies now buy Aloe vera gel in bulk from the United States to add it to their cosmetic products (Grindlay

& Reynolds, 1986).

Aloe vera may not be the "fountain of youth" to aged skin, and it most definitely will not produce the dramatic results that a face lift can. However, it is much easier to obtain than the "fountain of youth" and is far less expensive than a face lift. The important consideration when using Aloe vera cosmetic products is whether or not they contain the mannans known to produce the positive results reported in studies.

11

ALOE'S EFFECT ON OTHER HEALTH CONCERNS

Since Aloe has been looked upon as a curative of mythic propositions for much of recorded history, it is no wonder that there are dozens of health concerns that have been investigated. We have already examined those concerns that have received major research attention. However, there are many others that have received less attention. Research may discover positive effects in some of these lesser-studied applications that are of great significance to humankind.

CARDIOVASCULAR AND HEART RESEARCH

Heart disease is still the number one killer in the United States, but that terrible fact alone does not fully describe the effect of the disease. Most of those who ultimately die of heart disease have years of disability before they die. There is an enormous loss of productivity and enormous medical care costs associated with the disease.

And, most important, the loss of quality of life is devastating to those suffering heart disease and their love-ones. All large-scale studies of heart disease have shown beyond any doubt that the disease is one of the maladies most affected by lifestyle. Exercise and proper diet have been proven to lower the incidence and severity of the disease. All Americans know this to be true, and many have taken steps to gain more control of their health. For many reasons, including better treatment of hypertension, lower intake of alcohol, and less use of tobacco products, the per capita incidence of death from heart disease is down.

Still, humans are creatures of habit and old habits die very hard. Too much fat and too few fruits and vegetables in our diets, too little exercise, too much smoking and too much alcohol are all habits that many would like to keep. While we need to continue the massive public health campaign that has been going on for decades about the risk factors for heart disease, any regimen that can provide assistance needs to be explored.

That there is some evidence Aloe may be of assistance should not be surprising. One of the earliest and still most effective treatments for heart disease, digitalis, gets its active agent from the plant foxglove. "Our greatest killer is heart disease, but where would we be if the useful properties of foxglove had not been known empirically and then 'discovered' by a very astute botanist-physician several centuries ago? The answer should be obvious, since three million or more Americans daily take an extract from this plant to stay alive" (Lewis & Elvin-Lewis, 1977, 5).

HEART DISEASE, HYPERTENSION
AND ALOE VERA

One of the largest studies of the effect of Aloe on heart disease and hypertension was conducted by Dr. O.P. Agarwal in 1985. His massive study in Uttar Pradesh, India, covered 5,000 subjects over a five-year period. The patients were between the ages of 35 and 65, and all had evidence of heart disease in the form of ECG changes apart from effort angina (heart pain from vigorous exercise). All were screened for fasting blood sugar, post parandial blood sugar, total serum cholesterol, serum triglycerides, total lipids, and HDL cholesterol.

Some 3,000 of the patients were diabetics, 2,500 had a history of smoking, and 2,100 had hypertension, 800 of whom had moderate or severe hypertension. All 5,000 patients took 100 grams of fresh Aloe gel and 20 grams of Husk of Isabgol (a bulking agent) each day, mixed into their wheat flour bread. If the patient was taking medication for hypertension or otherconditions, they continued that course.

In his abstract, Dr. Agarwal notes, "[patients showed] a marked reduction in total serum cholesterol, serum triglycerides, fasting and post parandial blood sugar level in diabetic patients, total lipids and also an increase in HDL were noted. Simultaneously the clinical profile of these patients showed reduction in the frequency of anginal attacks and gradually, the drugs, like verapamil, ... were tapered. The patients most benefited were diabetics (without adding any antidiabetic drug).

The exact mechanism of the action of the above two substances is not known, but it appears, that probably they act by their high fibre contents. Both of these substances need further evaluation. The most interesting aspect of the study was that no untoward side effect was noted and all the 5,000 patients are surviving till date" (Agarwal, 1985, 485). Agarwal noted that most of the patients started responding after the second week from the start of the regimen. ECG changes started improving, and within three months to a year, all but 348 patients had normal ECG tracings even after being on a treadmill.

THE RESPIRATORY SYSTEM AND ASTHMA

As a folk medicine, Aloe is used to aid in the treatment of asthma and bronchitis by the native tribes of Java. They also use a mixture of Aloe and rose water to cure tuberculosis (Skousen).

Yagi (1987), found that a six-month oral administration of an Aloe extract showed efficacy for chronic bronchial asthmatics of various ages. In addition, Yagi found it significant that the extract was not efficacious for patients who had previously been administered corticosteroid.

As a topical agent, Aloe has been reported effective in treating respiratory tract disorders. A New Jersey physician (Thompson, 1991) has used a Beta (1,4) mannan Aloe gel for the treatment of post treatment epistaxis, nasal polyps, allergic rhinitis, non-specific rhinitis, and various skin inflammations. "In the respiratory tract, results are startling, taking place in hours to several days." Further, "The Carrington allantoin gotten from the Aloe vera plant seems to keep the admirable qualities of its root substances while in respiratory tract use, namely exerting a potent healing stimulus effect with virtually no discernible side effect or contraindications. Mucosal application of the gel seems to be far more rapid in promoting epithelialization of exposed bone following sinus surgery. The gel may be useful in accelerating healing of tracheotomies and mastoid cavity defects. It deserves significant testing in a variety of clinical uses where broad statistical data compilation is feasible. It may prove to be of inestimable importance" (Thompson, 1991, 119).

CIRRHOSIS AND HEPATITIS

A study (Oh et al., 1991) was conducted with seven patients diagnosed by hospitals as positive hepatitis and liver cirrhosis cases that had failed to show any improvement after courses of treatment that had continued in excess of two years. The patients/ average age was 47. They were not allowed to take any other liver-function medication during the study. Each patient was given an Aloe extract orally, and patients were interviewed each week. Liver-function tests were administered once per month. "Beginning approximately three months after the Aloe was first taken, the symptoms of indigestion in most patients began to show improvement, and the numerical values of liver-function tests (AST, ALT, Total bilirubin) were conducted on the patients, to compare their current symptoms with those present prior to the Aloe treatment; and it was noticed that significant medical effects had resulted since the commencement of the Aloe treatment" (Oh et al., 1991, 109).

AGING OF THE SKIN

As Danhof has pointed out (1991), many scientists now believe that a human life of some 120 years is not an unreasonable possibility. Death occurs at a much younger age because aging is "accelerated" by processes in the body and by external influences. Among the theories posed for internal processes that accelerate aging is that free radical generation associated with metabolic processes are most likely responsible for aging changes. This internal aging may be aggravated by exposure to actinic radiation (photo-aging). The skin in particular shows changes due to aging, becoming thinner, wrinkled, and less supple.

One of the naturally occurring agents which has shown the potential to retard skin aging is Aloe. Says Danof, "The amount of collagen in the skin can be measured by the presence of a marker substance, hydroxyproline. When oil-in-water (O/W) extracts were applied to guinea pig skin for six to sixteen weeks…the soluble collagen level, as denoted by the increase in hydroxyproline, was significantly increased—a remarkable potential anti-aging effect. Similar water-in oil (W/O) Aloe extracts were far less effective" (Danhof, 1991, 245).

OTHER IMPORTANT USES OF ALOE

Brown & Marcy (1991) interviewed 100 adults about their

use of botanical remedies. Over 100 different home remedies were identified, with most considered effective. Among the most frequently identified botanical was Aloe vera. Aloe has been known through time as one of the most versatile plants on Earth. Many of the most important uses have been discussed in detail in earlier chapters. There are, however, other uses that are significant as well.

ALOE AS A BACTERIOSTATIC

Studies have shown that Aloe is an effective bacteriostat. Lorenzetti et al. (1964) reported not only on the inhibition of bacterial growth in cell cultures, she also gave a brief account of the preparation needed to conserve the plant's effectiveness. "If tested immediately, the fresh juice exhibited a marked zone of inhibition...However the principle responsible for the inhibitory activity was found to be unstable. Preservatives such as sodium bisulfite, sodium benzoate, and methyl paraben were ineffective; however, the principle could be temporarily preserved by refrigeration and preserved for an even longer period by heating the juice for 15 minutes at 80 degrees. In all instances, the juice would gradually turn dark. Once the juice became dark, the inhibitory property was lost. If the juice that had been heated for 15 minutes at 80 degrees was freeze-dried, a buff-colored product resulted which was stable" (Lorenzetti, 1964, 1287).

USE OF ALOE IN DENTISTRY

Some of the early scientific exploratory work conducted in the 1970s and 1980s was done in the field of dentistry. Dr. Carrington, a long-time practitioner of dentistry in the Dallas/Fort Worth area, used Aloe extensively in his practice. Dental use as a periodontal dressing has been made of Aloe. One researcher conducted some extensive trials using Aloe as a dressing following periodontal surgery.

He "incorporated Aloe vera into two commercially available periodontal dressings. The dressings were placed into cell cultivations of epithelial and fibroblast cell lines. He discovered that higher dilutions of Aloe vera seemed to stimulate the growth rate of tissue culture cells when compared to the untreated controls.

Payne, in his topical use of Aloe vera following periodontal flap surgery, found that post operative pain was reduced more than with the normal saline control and swelling of tissues treated with Aloe vera was not as marked as the swelling of the control tissues. Also, the presence of a greater number of inflammatory cells and dilated vessels in the control tissue specimens, as compared to gingiva treated with Aloe vera, may indicate Aloe vera increases the rate of healing of periodontal surgical wounds" (Henry, 1978, 43).

ATHLETIC USES OF ALOE VERA

Aloe has been extensively used by athletes. Murray (1994) points to several who use it, including Spanky Stevens, an athletic trainer at the University of Texas who freezes Aloe gel, then uses it in conjunction with a methyl salicylate product and a cold hydrocollator to stop the peripheral bleeding and pain often associated with muscle strains and sprains. Piper (1983) reported that Stanford track coach Brooks Johnson used it extensively in his athletic program. "We clean off the area, crush some aspirin into a fine powder, then mix the two together and apply it to the injured area. The Aloe vera penetrates right through the skin, taking the aspirin directly into the bloodstream. We've found it works a lot faster that way because it's not diluted" (Piper, 1983, 46). Says Piper, "In short it's [Aloe] a medicine chest full of treatments in one package" (Piper, 1983, 46). Taylor-Donald (1992) reports that Ken Locker, trainer for the Dallas Cowboys, says that Aloe is effective on soft-tissue injuries, sprained ankles and thumbs, and for warming up sore muscles.

ALOE AS AN ADJUVANT

Finally, it has been shown that a Beta (1,4)-linked mannan extracted from Aloe has been proven effective as an adjuvant in vaccine preparations in the poultry industry. Chinnah et al. (1992) evaluated the mannans' use in a study on broiler chicks. The immune response to NDV [Newcastle disease virus] at 21 days post vaccination was significantly enhanced by the addition of the mannan. Carrington Laboratories has subsequently licensed the use of its acemannan to Solvay, an international manufacturer of veterinary pharmaceuticals, and millions of chicks are vaccinated each year.

Solvay International has full-page, color advertisements in the poultry industry trade journals promoting its "ACM-1" brand name for its enhanced vaccine. In large type, the ad states"The biggest thing to come along in years." ACM-1 has already revolutionized the economics of the broiler industry. Flock protection for Newcastle's, Merck's, and other diseases with use of this vaccine has been increased from 60-67 percent to 90-97 percent. The broilers gain more weight on less feed, T-cell lymphoma due to the Merck's virus is eliminated and no adverse events occured in 23 million birds vaccinated in the field studies. This was one of the largest biological studies ever conducted.

ALOE HEADS THE PARADE

Dr. McDaniel (1995) stated to me, "Scientific and medical skepticism, and criticism of our work crumbled with the results obtained in the Solvay adjuvant study. The paradigm for development of new medications was changing as we worked. The recognition of anti-cancer phytochemicals found in vegetables in studies at Johns Hopkins and Harvard Medical Schools followed by use of Taxol from the Pacific Yew tree in the treatment of cancer altered medical fashion. We started out as the subject of ridicule for researching Aloe as a source of a medication. Then one day we found that we were at the head of a parade of accomplishment while our critics were marching off to rain forests and digging into ancient manuscripts trying to find plants that might be a source for a new drug."

APPENDIXES
AND
BIBLIOGRAPHY

APPENDIX A

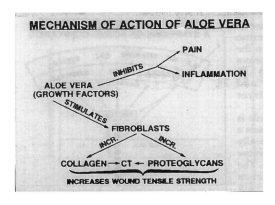

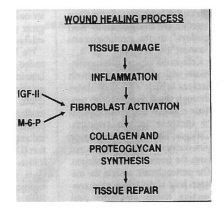

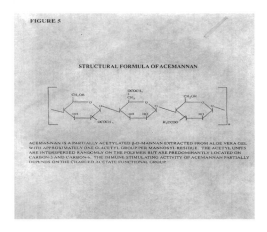

FIGURE 5

STRUCTURAL FORMULA OF ACEMANNAN

ACEMANNAN IS A PARTIALLY ACETYLATED β-D-MANNAN EXTRACTED FROM ALOE VERA GEL WITH APPROXIMATELY ONE O-ACETYL GROUP PER MANNOSYL RESIDUE. THE ACETYL UNITS ARE INTERSPERSED RANDOMLY ON THE POLYMER BUT ARE PREDOMINANTLY LOCATED ON CARBON-3 AND CARBON-6. THE IMMUNE STIMULATING ACTIVITY OF ACEMANNAN PARTIALLY DEPENDS ON THE CHARGED ACETATE FUNCTIONAL GROUP.

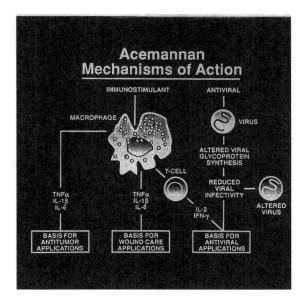

FIGURE 1

MACROPHAGE ACTIVATION-ORCHESTRATION OF CELLULAR AND HUMORAL DEFENSE AUGMENTED BY ACEMANNAN

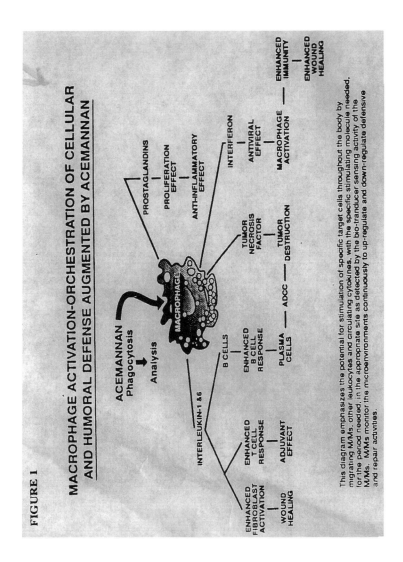

This diagram emphasizes the potential for stimulation of specific target cells throughout the body by migrating MMs, other leukocytes and circulating cytokines, with the specific stimulating molecule needed, for the period needed, in the appropriate site as detected by the bio-tranducer sensing activity of the MMs. MMs monitor the microenvironments continuously to up-regulate and down-regulate defensive and repair activities.

APPENDIX B

WHERE TO GET THE ALOE VERA PRODUCTS SIMILAR TO
THOSE MENTIONED IN THE RESEARCH IN THIS BOOK:

I.   MANNATECH INCORPORATED
     2010 North Highway 360
     Grand Prairie, TX 75050
     (214) 641-8829 • (800) 281-4469
     Fax (214) 641-8776 • Fax for Orders (800) 267-2722
     A. Man-Aloe™ – Oral tablets with the functional polymannans
found in fresh Aloe vera. Contains an effective lipid used to enhance the
bioavailability of the product and increase defense system support..
     B. Naturalizer™ – Advances the concept of skin care by utilizing
the amazing penetration qualities of Emu Oil to deliver Manapol® (the
functional component of fresh Aloe vera gel) deep into the layers of the
skin.
     C. Emprizone™ – An antiseptic hydrogel and Manapol® formula-
tion for the treatment of minor burns, scratches, cuts, insect bites and
other minor skin conditions.

II. THE CARING COMPANY
     17194 Preston Road, Suite 123-235
     Dallas, Texas 75248
     (800) 307-5858
     A. Carrisyn Hydrogel Wound Dressing™ – A hydrogel that main-
tains a moist wound environment, enhancing natural wound healing.
     B. Cara-Klenz™ – A cleanser which when sprayed on wounds re-
quires no scrubbing or rinsing. Can be applied to gauze for a moist wound
dressing
     C. Caraloe™ – A liquid drink or tablets which contain the active
ingredient of Aloe vera patented by Carrington Laboratories, Inc.

III. NEW LIFE NUTRICEUTICALS
     P. O. Box 996
     Boca Raton, FL 33429
     (407) 391-6844
     This company stocks the Aloe Vera Juice concentrate with active
ingredients recommended by Dr. Bruce Hedendal, producer and host of
"Health Hotline."

BIBLIOGRAPHY

Adams, Ruth. "Aloe Vera: Anti-Viral Agent." *Better Nutrition for Today's Living*. Vol. 54, No 4, April 1992, 21-26.

Ando, H., T. Asano, and N. Tsuchiva. "Cosmetics for Skin Care." *JPN*. Pat. 44,375, November 8, 1977.

Argawal, O. P. Presented at the Annual meeting of the American College of Angiology and the International College of Angiology, San Antonio, Texas. November 4, 1984.

Argawal, O. P. "Prevention of Atheromatous Heart Disease."

Angiology: The Journal of Vascular Disease. Vol 36, 1985, 485-492.

Aryayew, N.L., V. P. Filatov, and N.A. Puchkovskaya. Extract of Aloe: Scientific and Clinical Data." In Skousen, M. B. *The Aloe Vera Handbook*. Garden Grove, CA.

Ashley, F.L., B.J. O'Loughlin, R. Peterson, L. Fernandez, H. Stein, and A.N. Schwartz. "The Use of Aloe Vera in the Treatment of Thermal and Irradiation Burns in Laboratory Animals and Humans." *Plastic and Reconstructive Surgery*. Vol. 20, 1957, 383-396.

Balzarini, J. and S. Broder. "Principles of Antiviral Therapy for AIDS and Related Diseases." In De Clerq, E. (Ed.), *Clinical Use of Antiviral Drugs*. Boston: Martinue Nishoff Publishing, 1988, 361-385.

Barbul, Adrian. "Immune Aspects of Wound Repair." *Clinics in Plastic Surgery*. Vol. 17, No. 3, July 1990, 433-442.

Barnes, T.C. *American Journal of Botany*. 1967.

Beachy, Debra. "Nature's Pharmacy." *Houston Chronicle*. October 11, 1992, 1E.

Beppu, Hidehiko, Yohichi Nagamura, and Keisuke Fujita. "Hypoglycemic and Antidiabetic Effects of Aloe Arborsecens Miller var. natalensis Berger." Proceedings: International Congress of Phytotherapy. The Pharmaceutical Society of Korea, Aloe Research Foundation, U.S.A., October 16-17, 1991, Soeul, Korea.

Bland, Jeffrey. "Effect of Orally Consumed Aloe Vera Juice on Gastrointestinal Function in Normal Humans." *Preventive Medicine.* March/April, 1985, 135-139.

Blitz, Julian J., James W. Smith, and Jack R. Gerard. "Aloe Vera Gel in Peptic Ulcer Therapy: Preliminary Report." *Journal of the American Osteopathic Association.* Vol. 62, April, 1963, 731-735.

Borecky, L. V. Lacovic, and D. Blaskovic. "An Interferon-like Substance Induced by Mannans." *Acta Virol.* Vol. 11, 1967, 264-266.

Bowles, William B. "The Current Status of Aloe Vera Research." 1992.

Brown, J.S., and S.A. Marcy. "The Use of Botanicals for Health Purposes by Members of a Prepaid Health Plan." *Research in Nursing and Health.* Vol. 14, No. 5, October, 1991, 339-350.

Carrington Laboratories, Inc., "History of Acemannan Hydrogel." Company Profile. March, 1993.

Carrington Laboratories, Inc., "Helping the Body Fight Disease." Company Profile. April 15, 1993.

Cassidy, Catherine. "Aloe: A Bonus for Hair." *Fit*: "The Miracle Plant." Special Aloe Vera Reprint.

Cassidy, Catherine. "Save Face with Aloe." *Fit*: "The Miracle Plant" Special Aloe Vera Reprint.

Cera, Lee M., John P. Heggers, Martin C. Robson, and William J. Hagstrom. "The Therapeutic Efficacy of Aloe Vera Cream (Dermaide Aloe) in Thermal Injuries: Two Case Reports." *Journal of the American Animal Hospital Association.* Vol. 16, September/October 1980, 768-772.

Cera, Lee M., John P. Heggers, William J. Hagstrom, and Martin C. Robson. "Therapeutic Protocol for Thermally Injured Animals and Its Successful Use in an Extensively Burned Rhesus Monkey." *Journal of the American Animal Hospital Association.* Vol. 18, July/August 1982, 633-638.

Chapman, Daniel D., and Joseph J. Pittelli. "Double-Blind Comparison of Alophen with its Components for Cathartic Effects." *Current Therapeutic Research.* Vol. 16, No. 8, August, 1974, 817-820.

Chinnah, A.D., J.B. Kahlon, and M.C. Kemp. "Effect of Acemannan on the Function and Synthesis of HN and F Glycoproteins of Newcastle Disease Virus." Submitted to *Virology,* 1992.

Chinnah, Anthony D., Mirza A. Baig, Ian R. Tizard, and Maurice C. Kemp. "Antigen Dependent Adjuvant Activity of a Polydispersed B-(1,4)-Linked Acetylated Mannan (Acemannan). *Vaccine.* Vol. 10, No. 8, 1992, 551-557.

Clumeck, N. and P. Hermans. "Antiviral Drugs Other Than Zidovudine and Immunomodulating Therapies in Human Immunodeficiency Virus Infection." *Am. J. Med.* Vol. 85, 1988, 165-172.

Coats, Bill C. *The Silent Healer, A Modern Study of Aloe Vera.* 1984.

Collins, C.E., and Creston Collins. "Roentgen Dermatitis Treated with Fresh Whole Leaf of Aloe Vera." *American Journal of Roentgenology and Radium Therapy.* Vol 33, 1935, 396-397.

Combs, Frank C., and Max Scheer. "Roentgen Ray Dermatitis Treated with Ointment Containing Viosterol." *Archives of Dermatology and Syphilology.* Vol. 34, 1936, 901-903.

Crewe, J.E. "The External Uses of Aloes." *Minnesota Journal of Medicine.* Vol. 20, 1937, 538-539.

Danhof, Ivan E. "Aloe in Cosmetics – Does It Do Anything?" *Remarkable Aloe: Volume II.*

Danhof, Ivan E. "New Approach in the Treatment of Diabetic Foot Ulcers." *Cara: Medical Update.* Vol. 1, No. 1, July 1985.

Danhof, Ivan E. "Potential Reversal of Chronological and Photoaging of the Skin by Topical Application of Natural Substances." *Proceedings, International Congress of Phytotherapy.* October, 1991, 237-248.

Danhof, Ivan E. *Remarkable Aloe: Aloe Through the Ages.* Grand Prairie, Texas: Omnimedicus Press, 1987.

Danhof, Ivan E. "Some External Uses of Aloe." *Aloe Today.* Winter 1991/1992, 22-25.

Danhof, Ivan E. and Bill H. McAnalley. "Stabilized Aloe Vera: Effect on Human Skin Cells." *Drug and Cosmetic Industry.* August 1983, 52-54, 110.

Davis, Robert H., "Biological Activity of Aloe Vera." *Aloe Today.* Spring, 1993, 8-10.

Davis, Robert H., Joseph J. Di Donato, Glenn M. Hartman, and Richard C. Haas. "Anti-inflammatory and Wound Healing Activity of a Growth Substance in Aloe Vera." *Journal of the American Podiatric Medical Association.* Vol. 84, No. 2, February 1994, 77-81.

Davis Robert H., Joseph M. Kabbani, and Nicholas P. Maro. "Aloe Vera and Wound Healing." *Journal of the American Podiatric Medical Association.* Vol. 77, No. 4, April 1987, 165-169.

Davis, Robert H., Mark G. Leitner, and Joseph M. Russo. "Aloe Vera: A Natural Approach for Treating Wounds, Edema, and Pain in Diabetes." *Journal of the American Podiatric Medical Association.* Vol. 78, No. 2, February 1988, 60-68.

Davis, Robert H., M.G. Leitner, J.M. Russo, and M.E. Byrne. "Anti-inflammatory Activity of Aloe Vera Against a Spectrum of Irritants." *Journal of the American Podiatric Medical Association.* Vol. 79, No. 6, June 1989, 263-276.

Davis, Robert H., M.G. Leitner, J.M. Russo, and M.E. Byrne. "Wound Healing: Oral and Topical Activity of Aloe Vera." *Journal of the American Podiatric Medical Association.* Vol. 79, No. 11, 1989, 559-562.

Davis, Robert H. and Nicholas P. Maro. "Aloe Vera and Gibberellin: Anti-inflammatory Activity in Diabetes." *Journal of the American Podiatric Medical Association.* Vol. 79, No. 1, January 1989, 24-26.

Davis, Robert H., William L. Parker, and Douglas P. Murdoch. "Aloe Vera as a Biologically Active Vehicle for Hydrocortisone Acetate." *Journal of the American Podiatric Medical Association.* Vol. 81, No.1, January 1991, 1-9.

Davis, Robert H., William L. Parker, Richard T. Samson, Douglas, and P. Murdoch. "Isolation of a Stimulatory System in an Aloe Extract." *Journal of the American Podiatric Medical Association.* Vol. 81, No. 9, September 1991, 473-478.

Diller, I. C. "Degenerative Changes Induced in Tumors by S. Marcescens Polysaccharides." *Cancer Research.* Vol. 7, 1947, 605-626.

Edmonson, John N., Harry J. Long, Edward T. Creagan, Stephen Frutak, Stephen A. Sherwin, and Myron N. Chang. "Phase II Study of Recombinant Gamma-Interferon in Patients with Advanced Nonosseous Sarcomas." *Cancer Treatment Reports.* Vol. 71, No. 2, February 1987, 211-213.

Fine, Archie, and Samuel Brown. "Cultivation and Clinical Application of Aloe Vera Leaf." *Radiology.* Vol. 31, 1938, 735-736.

Finn, Peter. "New AIDS Drug Faces Lengthy Approval Path." *Fort Worth Star-Telegram.* June 11, 1994.

Flagg, J. "Aloe Vera Gel in Dermatological Preparations." *American Perfumer.* Vol. 74, 1959, 27.

Fujita, Keisuke, Ryoh Teradaira, and Toshiharu Hagatsu. "Bradykininase Activity of Aloe Extract." *Biochemical Pharmacology.* Vol. 25, 1976, 205.

Fulton, James E. "The Stimulation of Postdermabrasion Wound Healing with Stabilized Aloe Vera Gel-Polyethylene Oxide Dressing." *J. Dermatol. Surg. Oncol.* Vol. 16, 1990, 460-467.

Ghannam, N., M. Kingston, I.A. Al-Meshaal, M. Tariq, N.S. Parman, and N. Woodhaus. "The Antidiabetic Activity of Aloes: Preliminary Clinical and Experimental Observations." *Hormone Research.* Vol. 24, 1986, 288-294.

Gjerstad, G. "An Appraisal of the Aloe Vera Juice." *American Perfumer and Cosmetics.* Vol. 84, 1969, 43-46.

Gjerstad, G. and T.D. Riner. "Current Status of Aloe as a Cure-All." *American Journal of Pharmacy.* Vol. 140, 1968, 58-64.

Goldstein, David and John Laszlo. "Interferon Therapy in Cancer: From Imaginon to Interferon." *Cancer Research.* Vol. 46, September 1986, 4315-4329.

Grander, D., K. Oberg, M.L. Lundqvist, Janson E. Tiensuu, B. Eriksson, and S. Einhorn. "Interferon-induced Enhancement of 2', 5'-oligoadenylate Synthetase in Mid-Gut Carcinoid Tumors." *Lancet.* Vol. 2, 1990, 337-340.

Green, Gordon. "Dallas Morbidity Report: AIDS-Related Health Frauds." *Dallas Medical Journal.* Vol. 75, 1989, 13.

Greene, Warner C."AIDS and the Immune System." *Scientific American.* September 1993, 99-105.

Grindlay, Douglas and T. Reynolds. "The Aloe Vera Phenomenon: A Review of the Properties and Modern Uses of the Leaf Parenchyma Gel." *Journal of Ethnopharmacology.* Vol. 16, 1986, 117-151.

Hanley, Denice C., William A.B. Soloman, Barry Saffran, and Robert H. Davis. "The Evaluation of Natural Substances in the Treatment of Adjuvant Arthritis." *Journal of the American Podiatry Association.* Vol. 72, No 6, June, 1982, 275-284.

Harris, Cheryl, Ken Pierce, Glen King, Kenneth M. Yates, John Hall and Ian Tizard. "Efficacy of Acemannan in Treatment of Canine and Feline Spontaneous Neoplasms." *Molecular Biotherapy.* Vol. 3, December 1991, 207-213.

Hasenclever, H.G. and W.O. Mitchell. "Immunochemical Studies on Polysaccharides of Yeasts." *J. Bact.* Vol. 93, 1964, 763-771.

Hazelton, Lloyd W. "The Influence of Aloe and Podophyllum on the Flow of Heptic Bile in the Dog." *Journal of the American Pharmaceutical Association.* Vol. 31, 1942, 53-56.

Heggers, John P. "Beneficial Effects of Aloe in Wound Healing." Proceedings: International Congress of Phytotherapy. The Pharmaceutical Society of Korea, Aloe Research Foundation, U.S.A. October 16-17, 1991.

Heggers, John P., and Martin C. Robson. "Prostaglandins and Thromboxane." *Critical Care Clinics.* Vol. 1, No. 1, March 1985, 59-77.

Hennessee, Odus, M., and Bill R. Cook. *Aloe: Myth-Magic Medicine.* Lawton, OK: Universal Graphics, 1989.

Henry, Ray. "An Updated Review of Aloe Vera." *Cosmetics and Toiletries.* Vol. 94, June 1978, 42-46.

Hikino, H., M. Takahashi, M. Marakami, C. Konno, Y. Mirin, M. Darikura, and T. Hayashi. "Isolation and Hypoglycemic Activity of Arborans A and B, Blycans of Aloe arborescens Mill. Var. natalensis Leaves." *International Journal of Crude Drug Research.* Vol. 24, No. 4, 1986, 183-186.

Ikawa, Myoshi, and Carl Niemann. "Further Observations on the Behavior of Carbohydrates in 79% Sulfuric Acid." *Archives of Biochemistry and Prophysics.* Vol. 3161, 1951, 70-71.

Inanishi, Ken'ichi. "Aloctin A, An Active Substance of Aloe arborescens Miller as an Immunomodulator." *Phytotherapy Research.* Vol. 7, 1993, 20-22.

Investigator Brochure: Acemannan (Carrisyn®) for Injection: AIDS." Carrington Laboratories, Inc., Irving, Texas, July 22, 1992.

James, John S. *AIDS Treatment News.* Berkley, California: Celestial Arts, 1989.

Johnson, Alice R., Anita C. White, and Bill McAnalley. "Comparison of Common Topical Agents for Wound Treatment: Cytotoxicity for Human Fibroblasts in Culture." *Wounds.* Vol. 1, 1989, 186-192.

Kahlon, Jasbir B., Maurice C. Kemp, Robert H. Carpenter, Bill H. McAnalley, H. Reg McDaniel, and William M. Shannon. "Inhibition of AIDS Virus Replication by Acemannan In Vitro." *Molecular Biotherapy.* Vol. 3, September, 1991, 127-135.

Kahlon, Jasbir B., Maurice C. Kemp, Ni Yawei, Robert H. Carpenter, William M. Shannon, and Bill H. McAnalley. "In Vitro Evaluation of the Synergistic Antiviral Effects of Acemannan in Combination with Azidothymidine and Acyclovir." *Molecular Biotherapy.* Vol. 3, December 1991, 214-223.

Kaufman, Theodor, Noam Kalderon, Yehuda Ullmann, and Joseph Berger. "Aloe Vera Gel Hindered Wound Healing of Experimental Second-Degree Burns: A Quantitative Controlled Study." *Journal of Burn Care Rehabilitation.* Vol. 9, No. 2, March/April 1988, 156-159.

Kemp, M.C., J.B. Kahlon, and A.D. Chinnah. "In Vitro Evaluation of the Antiviral Effects of Acemannan on the Replication and Pathogenesis of Hiv -1 and Other Enveloped Viruses: Modification of the Processing of Glycoprotein Precursors." Proceedings of the Third International Conference on Antiviral Research. 1990.

Kemp, M.C., J.B. Kahlon, A.D. Chinnah, R.H. Carpenter, B.H. McAnalley, H.R. McDaniel, and W.M. Shannon. "In Vitro Evaluation of the Antiviral Effects of Acemannan on the Replication and Pathogenesis of HIV-1 and Other Enveloped Viruses: Modification of the Processing of Glycoprotein Precursors." *AIDS.* Abstract #84, page 83.

Kent, C.M. Aloe Vera. Arlington, VA: Carol Miller Kent, 1979.

King, Glen and Ken Pierce. "Management and Treatment of Canine and Feline Fibrosarcoma with Acemannan: Follow-up Report." Carrington Research and Development Document # 8306.1 June 1, 1992.

Kivett, William F. "Aloe Vera for Burns." *Plastic and Reconstructive Surgery.* Vol. 83, No. 1, January, 1989, 195.

Lackovic, Vladimir, Ladislar Borecky, Dobroslav Sikl, Ladislav Masler, and Stefan Bauer. "Stimulation of Interferon Production by Mannans." *Proceedings of the Society for Experimental Biology and Medicine.* Vol. 134, 1970, 874-879.

Leung, Albert Y. "Aloe Vera in Cosmetics." *Excelsa.* Vol. 8, 1978, 65-68.

Lewis, Walter H., and Memory Elvin-Lewis. *Medical Botany: Plants Affecting Man's Health.* John Wiley & Sons, NY, 1977.

The Local Action of Aloes on Regeneration" *The Journal of American Veterinary Medical Association.* October, 1941.

Lorenzetti, Lorna J., Rupert Salisbury, Jack L. Beal, and Jack N. Baldwin. "Bacteriostatic Property of Aloe Vera." *Journal of Pharmaceutical Sciences.* Vol. 53, 1964, 1287.

Loveman, Adolph B. "Leaf of Aloe Vera in Treatment of Roentgen Ray Ulcers." *Archives of Dermatology and Syphilology.* Vol. 36, 1937, 838-843.

Lushbaugh, C.C., and D.B. Hale. "Experimental Acute Radiodermatitis Following Beta Radiation." *Cancer.* 1953, 65.

Lushaugh, C.C., and D.B. Hale. "Experimental Acute Radiodermatitis Following Beta Irradiation: V. Histopathological Study of the Mode of Action of Therapy with Aloe Vera." *Cancer.* Vol. 6, No. 4, July 1953, 690-698.

McAnalley, B.H. Carrington Laboratories, Inc., Process or Preparation of Aloe Products, Products Produced Thereby and Compositions Thereof, Reg. Pat. No. 4,735,935, April 5, 1988.

McAnalley, Bill H., and D. Eric Moore. "Wound Cleanser." United States Patent #5,284,833, February 8, 1994.

McAnnalley, Bill H. "Ulceroprotection by Aloe Extract in the Reserpine-Induced Ulcer Model in the Rat." Carrington Research and Development Document No. 6015, 1989.

McCauley, Robert L., David N. Hing, Martin C. Robson, and John P. Heggers. "Frostbite Injuries: A Rational Approach Based on the Pathophysiology." Unpublished, Martin C. Robson, Section of Plastic and Reconstructive Surgery, The University of Chicago, 950 E. 59th St., Chicago IL 60637.

McCauley, Robert L., John P. Heggers, and Martin C. Robson. "Frostbite: Methods to Minimize Tissue Loss." *Postgraduate Medicine*. Vol. 88, No. 8, December 1990, 67-77.

McDaniel, Reginald. Interview at Emprise International. Grand Prairie, TX, May 1995.

McDaniel, Reginald. "The Aloe Mystery is Solved: Manapol Did It!" Unpublished Paper, 1994.

McDaniel, H. Reg. "Carrington's Aloe Story." Cassette Tape. Dallas, TX: Fisher Institute for Medical Research, 1994.

McDaniel, H. Reg, Bill H. McAnalley, and Robert Carpenter. "The Basic Science and Principles for the Use of Acemannan in Clinical Medicine." Pre-publication Manuscript, 1994.

McDaniel, H. Reg, Sue Perkins, and B.H. McAnalley. "A Clinical Pilot Study Using Carrisyn™ in the Treatment of Acquired Immunodeficiency Syndrome (AIDS). *American Journal of Clinical Pathology*. October, 1987.

Magness, Bruce. "Aloe Vera – Nature's Perfect Healer." *Aloe Today*. Aloecorp, 2809 E. Grimes, Harlingen, TX 78550, Summer, 1993, 27-29.

Mandeville, Frederick B. "Aloe Vera in the Treatment of Radiation Ulcers of Mucous Membranes." *Radiology*. Vol. 32, 1939, 598-599.

Marshall, G.D., A.S. Gibbons, and L.S. Parnell. "Human Cytokines Induced by Acemannan." Abstract #619. *Journal of Allergy and Chemical Immunology.* Vol. 91, No. 619, 1993, 295.

Morison, S.E. *Journals and Other Documents on the Life and Voyages of Christopher Columbus.* New York, 1963.

Mosby's Medical Dictionary. Baltimore: C.V. Mosby Company. 1990.

Murray, Frank. "Therapy and Treatment with Aloe Vera." *Better Nutrition For Today's Living.* March, 1994, 52-55.

Network Update. "First North American Trial of Acemannan Begins in January." Vol 1, No 5, Nov/Dec, 1990.

News Release. "Carrington Laboratories Encouraged by Results from Canadian Clinical Trial of Oral Acemannan in AIDS Patients." December 23, 1992.

Obata, Masafumi, Shosuke Ito, Hidehiko Beppu and Keisuke Fujita. "Mechanism of Anti-Inflammatory and Anti-Thermal Burn Action of Aloe Arborescens Mill. Var. Natalensis Berger." Proceedings: International Congress of Phytotherapy. The Pharmaceutical Society of Korea, Aloe Research Foundation, U.S.A., October 16-17, 1991, Soeul, Korea.

Odes, H. S. , and Z. Madar. "A Double-Blind Trial of a Celandin, Aloe Vera and Psyllium: A Laxative Preparation in Adult Patients with Constipation." *Digestion.* Vol. 49, 1991, 65-71.

Oh, You-Jin, Woong-Yang Park, Kwan-Hoi Kim, Jin-Tae Hong, and Yeo-Pyo Yun. "Effect of Aloe Vera Linne and Aloe Arborescens Miller Mixture of the Hepatitis and Liver Cirrhosis Patients." Proceedings, International Congress of Phytotherapy. October 16, 1991, 107-116.

Parnell, L. and Ian R. Tizard. "Accelerated Wound Healing in Guinea Pigs Treated with a Complex Carbohydrate." Presented at the European Tissue Repair Society. Malmo, Sweden, August 26, 1992.

Pedersen, Niels C., and Jeffrey E. Barlough. "Clinical Overview of Feline Immunodeficiency Virus." *Journal of the American Veterinary Medicine Association.* Vol. 199, No. 10, November 15, 1991, 1298-1304.

Pelley, R. P. "Aloe Quality Control: Certification of Nam Yang Aloe Company Products." *Aloe Today*, Autumn-Winter, 1990-1991, 12-15.

Peng, S.Y., J. Norman, G. Curtin, D. Corrier, H.R. McDaniel, and D. Busbee. "Decreased Mortality of Norman Murine Sarcoma in Mice Treated with the Immunomodulator, Acemannan™." *Molecular Biotherapy.* Vol. 3, June 1991, 79-87.

Physicians Desk Reference. Montvale, NJ: Medical Economics Data Production Company. 1994.

Piper, Chuck, with Kevin Baxter. "Treating Injuries with Aloe Vera." *Runner's World*, January, 1983, 44-46.

Pullin, Dennis. "Sports Medicine: A Meeting of Folklore and Science." *City Fitness Magazine.* September,1994.

Ray Dirks Research. "The Acemannan Report." *Health Consciousness.* Vol. 13, No. 1, 1992, 43-46.

Rector-Page, Linda G. *Healthy Healing: An Alternative Healing Reference.* Healthy Healing Publications, 1992.

Robson, Martin C., Aileen Jellma, John P. Heggers, and William J. Hagstrom. "Care of the Healed Wound: A Prospective Randomized Study." American Burn Association Twelfth Annual Meeting Report, March 27, 1980, 94-95.

Robson, M.C., R.C. Murphy, and J.P. Heggers. "A New Explanation for the Progressive Tissue Loss in Electrical Injury." *Plastic and Reconstructive Surgery.* Vol. 73, 1984, 431-437.

Rodriguez-Bigas, Miguel, Norma I.P. Cruz, and Albert Suarez. "Comparative Evaluation of Aloe Vera in the Management of Burn Wounds in Guinea Pigs." *Plastic and Reconstructive Surgery.* Vol. 81, No. 1, March 1988, 386-389.

Rowe, Tom D., B.K. Lovell, and Lloyd M. Parks. "Further Observations on the Use of Aloe Vera Leaf in the Treatment of Third Degree X-Ray Reactions." *Journal of the American Pharmaceutical Association.* Vol. 30, 1941, 266-269.

Rowe, T.D., and L.M. Parks. "A Phytochemical Study of Aloe Vera Leaf." *Journal of the American Pharmaceutical Asssociation,* Vol. 39, 1939, 262-265.

Rubinstein, A., C. Pierce, and Z. Bloombearden. "Rapid Healing of Diabetic Foot Ulcers with Continuous Subcutaneous Insulin Infusion." *American Journal of Medicine.* Vol. 75, 1983, 161.

Schechter, Steven R. "Aloe Vera Produces Anti-Inflammatory, Immune Strenghtening Effects on Skin." *Let's Live.* December 1994, 50-52.

Sener, B. and F. Bingol. "Screening of Natural Sources for Antiinflammatory Acitvity: Review." *Int. J. Crude Drug Res.* Vol. 26, No. 4, 1988, 197-207.

Sheets, Mark A., Beverly A. Unger, Gene F. Giggleman, and Ian R. Tizard. "Studies of the Effect of Acemannan on Retrovirus Infections: Clinical Stabilization of Feline Leukemia Virus-Infected Cats." *Molecular Biotherapy.* Vol. 3, March 1991, 41-45.

Sherry, Michael M. *Confronting Cancer: How to Care for Today and Tomorrow.* New York: Insight Books, 1994.

Ship, Arthur George, "Is Topical Aloe Vera Plant Mucus Helpful in Burn Treatment?" *Journal of the American Medical Association.* Vol. 238, No. 16, October 17, 1977, 1770.

Skousen, M. B. *The Aloe Vera Handbook.* Garden Grove, CA.

Stachow, A., B. Sawicka, and D. Kieniewska. "Hydrozyproline Determination for Evaluation of the Effect of Cosmetic Cream on Guinea Pig Skin Collagen. *Aerzl Kosmetol.* Vol. 14, 1984, 376-377, 380.

Strickland, Faith M., Ronald P. Pelley, Donald Hill, and Margaret L. Kripke. "Reversal of UVB-Induced Suppression of Contact Sensitivity in C3H Mice by Topical Administration of Aloe Barbadensis Gel Extracts." *Photochemistry and Photobiology.* Vol. 55, No 6, 1992.

Swaim, Steven F., Kay P. Riddell, and John A. McGuire. "Effects of Topical Medications on the Healing of Open Pad Wounds in Dogs." *Journal of the American Animal Hospital Association.* Vol. 28, 1992, 499-506.

Taylor-Donald, Laurie. "Aloe: The Miracle of Aloe Vera." *Fit:* "The Miracle Plant" Special Aloe Vera Reprint.

Thompson, James E. "Topical Use of Aloe Vera Derived Allantoin Gel in Otolaryngology." *Ear, Nose, and Throat Journal.* Vol. 70, No. 2, 1991, 119.

Thompson, Rita. *Lupus, Aloe Vera, and Me.* Toledo, Ohio.

Times Picayune. "Aloe Drug May Mimic AZT Without Toxicity." 1989.

Tizard, Ian R. "Carbohydrates, Immune Stimulating." Roitt, Ivan M. and Peter J. Delves, Eds. *Encyclopedia of Immunology.* London: Academic Press, 1992.

Tizard, Ian R. "The Effect of Acemannan on the Healing of Wounds in Experimental Animals." Presented at the International Symposium on Wound Healing and Wound Management. New Orleans, Louisiana. October 10, 1992.

Tizard, Ian. Use of Immunomodulators as an Aid to Clinical Management of Feline Leukemia Virus-Infected Cats. *Journal of American Veterinary Medical Association.* Vol. 199, No. 10, November 15, 1991, 1482-1485.

Tizard, Ian R., Robert H. Carpenter, Bill H. McAnalley, and Maurice C. Kemp. "The Biological Activities of Mannans and Related Complex Carbohydrates." *Molecular Biotherapy.* Vol. 1, No. 6, 1989, 290-296.

Tsuda, H., K. Matsumoto, M. Ito, I. Hirono, K. Kawai, H. Beppu, K. Fujita, and M. Nagoo. "Inhibitory Effect of Aloe arborescens Miller var. natalensis Berger (Kidachi Aloe) on Induction of Preneoplastic Focal Lesions in the Rat Liver." *Phytotherapy Research*. Vol. 7, 1993, 43-47.

Waller, Todd."Designing a Personal Care Product Using Aloe Vera." *Aloe Today*. Spring/Summer, 1992, 6-9.

Weerts, D., S. DeWit, M. Gerard, F. Rahir, J. Jonckheere and N. Clumeck. "A Phase II Study of Carrisyn® (Acemannan) Aloe and with AZT Among Symptomatic and Asymptomatic HIV Patients." Presented at the Sixth International Conference on AIDS. San Francisco, California. June 20-21, 1990. Retrospective Analysis Dated June, 1992.

Winters, W.D., R. Benavides, and W.J. Clouse. "Effects of Aloe Extract on Human Normal and Tumor Cells in Vitro." *Economic Biology*. Vol. 35, No. 1, 1981, 89-95.

Womble, D. and J.H. Helderman. "Enhancement of Allo-Responsiveness of Human—Lymphocytes by Acemannan (Carrisyn®)." *International Journal of Immunopharmacology*. Vol. 10, 1988, 967-974.

Womble, D. and J.H. Helderman. "The Impact of Acemannan on the Generation and Function of Cytotoxic T-Lymphocytes." *Immunopharmacology and Immunotoxicology*. Vol. 14, Nos 1 and 2, 1992, 63-77.

Wright, Carroll S. "Aloe Vera in the Treatment of Roentgen Ulcers and Telangiectasis." *Journal of the American Medical Association*. April 18, 1936, 1363-1364.

Yagi, Akira. "Effect of Amino Acids in Aloe Extract on Phagocytosis by Peripheral Neutrophil in Adult Bronchial Asthma." *Japan Journal of Allergology*. Vol. 36, No. 12, 1987, 1094-1101.

Yates, K.M., L.J. Rosenberg, C.K. Harris, D.C. Bronstad, G.K. King, G.A. Biehle, B. Walker, C.R. Ford, J.E. Hall, and I.R. Tizard. "Pilot Study of the Effect of Acemannan in Cats Infected with Feline Immunodeficiency Virus." *Veterinary Immunology and Immunopathology*. Vol. 35, 1992, 177-189.

Yarchoan, R., H. Mitsuya, and S. Broder. "Strategies for Combination Therapy of HIV Infection." *Journal of AIDS.* Vol. 3, 1990, S99-S103.

Zawahry, M.E., M. Rashad Hegazy, and M. Helal. "Use of Aloe in Treating Leg Ulcers and Dermatoses." *International Journal of Dermatology.* Vol. 12, 1973, 68-73.

INDEX

All inquiries and orders for:

THE MIRACLE IN ALOE VERA: THE FACTS ABOUT POLYMANNANS,
or
BOUNTIFUL HEALTH, BOUNDLESS ENERGY, BRILLIANT YOUTH: THE FACTS ABOUT DHEA

Should be addressed to:

CHARIS PUBLISHING CO.

P. O. Box 740607 • Dallas, Texas 75374
(214) 342-1137 • Fax (214) 739-6644 ext. 8

SINGLE BOOK PRICE...................................... **$12.95 EACH**
TWO TO 20 COPIES .... **9.95 EACH**
OVER 20 COPIES .... **8.95 EACH**
100+ COPIES .... **7.95 EACH**

Please send _____ copies @ _____ $ _____

Texas residents add 8.25% tax .... $ _____

Shipping & Handling (See Below) .... $ _____

1 Book – $2.25
2 - 20 Books – $1 per book
Over 20 Books – 70¢ per book

TOTAL AMOUNT ENCLOSED $ _____

SHIPPING INFORMATION:

NAME _____

ADDRESS _____

CITY, STATE, ZIP _____

HOME PHONE _____

WORK PHONE _____

120